Better Food for Dogs

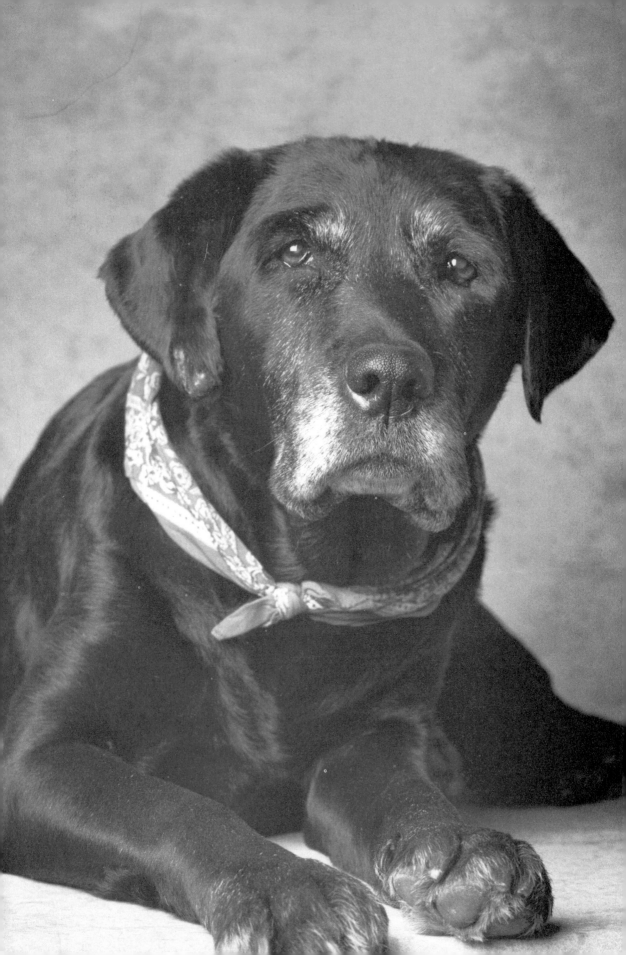

Better Food for Dogs

A complete cookbook & nutrition guide

DAVID BASTIN, JENNIFER ASHTON
and DR. GRANT NIXON, D.V.M.

Robert
ROSE

For complete cataloguing information, see page 214.

Disclaimer
The nutritional information and the recipes in this book have been reviewed by an
independent professional animal nutrition consultant. To the best of our knowledge
they are safe and nutritious for ordinary use with dogs. For those people who have dogs
with food or other allergies, or who have dogs who have special food requirements or
health issues, please read the suggested contents of each recipe carefully and determine
whether or not they may create a problem for your dog. All nutritional information
and recipes are used at the risk of the reader/purchaser.

We cannot be responsible for any hazards, loss or damage that may occur to your dog
as a result of any nutritional information or recipe use.

For those dogs with special needs, allergies, requirements or health problems or, in the
event of any doubt, please contact your dog's veterinary adviser prior to the use of any
recipe. Every dog may be different in its nutritional needs which should therefore be
checked with your dog's veterinarian as to its use and continued use.

These recipes are intended for dogs only and should not be used for any other purpose.

Design & Production: PageWave Graphics Inc.
Editor: Judith Finlayson
Copy Editor: Christina Anson Mine
Recipe Editor: Jennifer MacKenzie
Black & white photography: Karen Perlmutter
Color photography: Siberian Husky © iStock.com/tunart; Yorkshire Terrier ©
iStock.com/Joanna Pecha; Golden Retriever © iStock.com/Carrie Bottomley; Basset
Hound © iStock.com/Stockphoto4u; Weimaraner (Retriever) © iStock.com/Eric Isselée;
Collie © iStock.com/daneger; Scottish Terrier © iStock.com/Natallia Yaumenenka;
Chihuahua © iStock.com/Marcin Pikula; Dalmation © iStock.com/daneger; Australian
Shepherd © iStock.com/Eric Isselée; Dog with Turquoise Dish © iStock.com/CountryStyle
Photography; Mixed Breed © iStock.com/Eric Isselée; Boston Terrier © iStock.com/
Rhys Hastings; Mixed Breed © iStock.com/Eric Isselée; American Cocker Spaniel
© iStock.com/Vladimir Mucibabic; Poodle © iStock.com/Eric Isselée

Cover Image: Larry Williams/corbis/firstlight.ca

We acknowledge the financial support of the Government of Canada through the
Book Publishing Industry Development Program (BPIDP) for our publishing activities.

Published by: Robert Rose Inc.
120 Eglinton Ave. E., Suite 800, Toronto, Ontario, Canada M4P 1E2
Tel: (416) 322-6552 Fax: (416) 322-6936
www.robertrose.ca

Printed and bound in Canada
9 10 11 12 13 14 15 16   MP   19 18 17 16 15 14 13 12

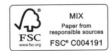

· ·

This book is dedicated to dogs everywhere.
Please remember, some of the greatest friends you'll ever have
are waiting to be adopted at your local animal shelter.

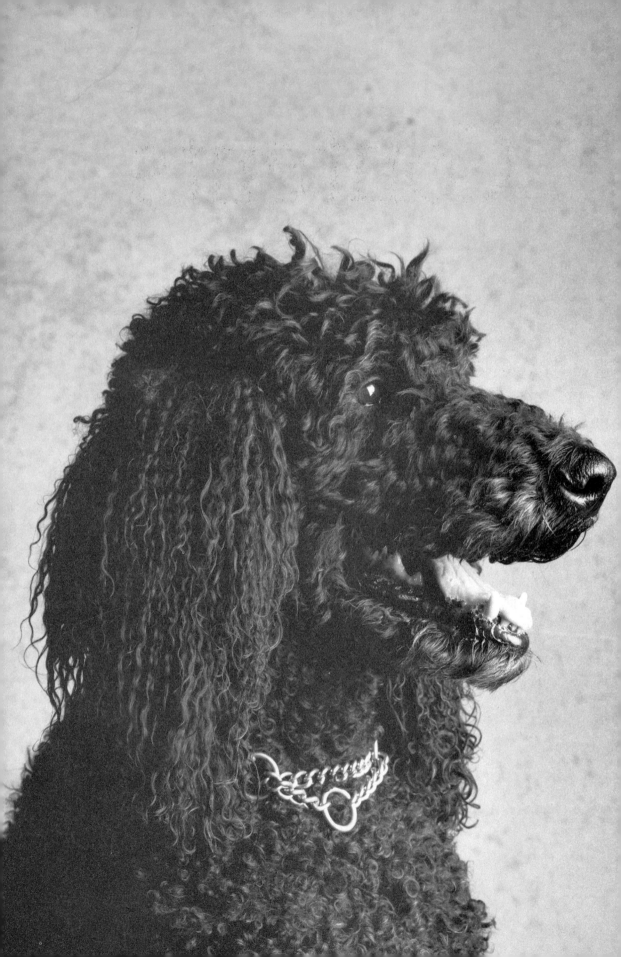

Contents

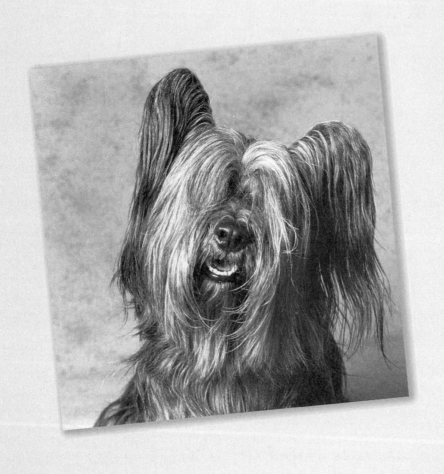

Acknowledgments

DAVID AND JENNIFER WOULD LIKE TO EXTEND THEIR deepest gratitude to the following people and dogs — without them, this book would never have been written.

Harris, Zoee, Marley, Buffett and Dylan for being the very special dogs that they are. The Notlobs for providing the impetus. Mike and Lynn McCrady for their support. Beryl and Doug for believing in them. Carey, Kelly and the Boyz at Lucid Distributors for helping to make their cookies so famous. Their other distributors and the many great stores that provide their yummy cookies to their customers. Diane, David, Bournville and Susie for taking Licks and Wags to the United Kingdom and Europe. All of their wonderful, four-legged, furry customers and their significant humans who buy their cookies. Dr. Grant Nixon for his enthusiasm and for providing such compassionate veterinary care to their dogs. Gary and the crew at Video Innovation Productions. Everyone at "The Vicki Gabereau Show" for letting them cook for them, for being such gracious hosts and for giving Dylan his national television debut. Arden's husband for seeing them on television. Arden for pulling for them. Bob for giving them the opportunity and trusting them to write this book. Jan for answering so many of their questions and not getting call display. Special thanks to George! Jennifer for ensuring that their recipes met the highest standards of exactness and Tina, outstanding chief of the grammar police. The team at PageWave Graphics — Andrew, Joseph and Kevin — for designing such a great-looking book. Judith for doing such a great job of eloquently macheteing her way through the jungle that was their manuscript and turning it into the great book that it is. And last, but not least, their families for their love, patience and support.

Grant would like to thank his loving, supportive wife, Wendy, and his three beautiful children, Lauren, Gregory and Daniel. He would also like to thank with love and pats his own special dog, Otis, and his many furry patients that have offered him inspiration and insight through the completion of this book.

Introduction

MOST DOGS — AT LEAST THE FORTUNATE ONES — ARE well loved and well cared for by their significant humans. People recognize their canine companions' value as family members, life-enhancers and educators and want them to have the healthiest — and longest — lives possible. Providing the best nutrition plays an important role in achieving this result. The problem is, most of us aren't nutritionists. Moreover, there are so many conflicting opinions about dogs' dietary needs that determining what to feed your dog can be an overwhelming challenge.

Better Food for Dogs is designed to guide you through the differing dietary approaches and provide you with all the information you need to feed your adult dog the most-nutritious food possible. We navigated this minefield ourselves, not only because we wanted to feed our dogs the highest-quality food achievable, but also because we wanted to provide our clients with the best possible advice on dogs' dietary needs and be able to recommend the most nutritious products. Grant is a veterinarian and David and Jennifer own *Licks and Wags, Ltd.*, a dog cookie company. After years of research, we've concluded that a natural, home-prepared diet is one of the best investments you can make in your dog's health. We wrote this book because we felt compelled to share what we had so painstakingly learned.

Chapter 1 covers a wide range of diet-related topics, from the relationship between diet and health to raw-food diets (which we don't advocate, for reasons we explain). In Chapter 2, you'll find an explanation of the basic principles that underlie our diet, as well as information on dogs' energy requirements and the nutrients they need. We have not provided a diet for puppies, as puppies have very specific nutritional needs. However, we have included basic information that will help you get your puppy off to a healthy start. Chapter 3 discusses some issues related to diet, such as allergic reactions and toxic foods, as well as the additional support your dog will need to achieve optimum health. Chapters 4, 5, and 6 contain all the recipes, from basic everyday meals to gourmet dinners to special cookie treats. The final chapter provides information on adding the supplements necessary to ensure that your dog receives the full range of essential nutrients.

We hope you will find the information in *Better Food for Dogs* helpful in improving the quality of your dog's life. After switching to a home-prepared diet, we have seen amazing results, not only with our own dogs but with many of our clients' dogs, as well. By feeding your dog wholesome and unprocessed foods, you will be allowing him/her to share in the tastes, variety and health benefits that human family members already enjoy. We encourage you to enjoy sharing mealtime with your dog — it can be a rewarding and mutually beneficial experience.

David Bastin
Jennifer Ashton
Dr. Grant Nixon, D.V.M.

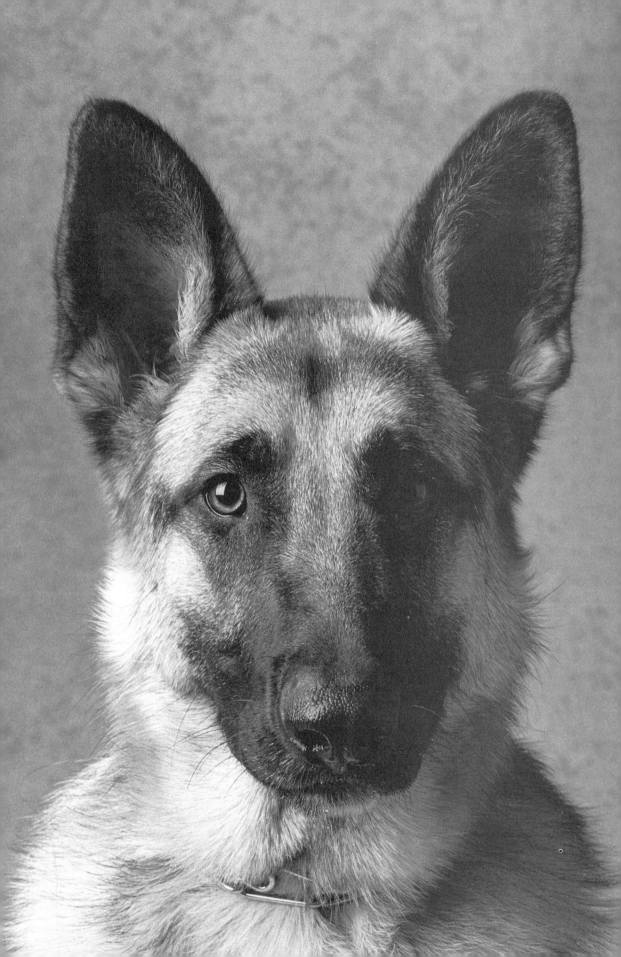

The Canine Diet

MADDY — 14-MONTH-OLD GERMAN SHEPHERD

Dogs and Humans: Similar yet Different

HUMANS AND CANINES HAVE BEEN CLOSELY CONNECTED throughout their mutual histories. While we don't fully understand how, or why, our two species came together, the bond between human beings and dogs is deep and complex. Although both species have benefited from this unique relationship, domestication has altered dogs in many ways, including their ability to choose what they eat.

Dogs are physically built to hunt for animal sources of protein, a natural behavior that has been increasingly discouraged as civilization has advanced. But even though they belong to the carnivore group, which means they are meat eaters, dogs aren't obligate carnivores, like cats, because they are able to survive by eating plants as well as animals. This ability to survive on a varied diet also classifies dogs, like humans, as omnivores — a similarity that has enabled them to live easily alongside humans.

Diet and Health

Good nutrition is imperative for good health. As the old saying goes, "An ounce of prevention is worth a pound of cure." This is true for dogs as well as people. A healthy diet can help to promote longevity and improve your dog's quality of life. It may also help to prevent disease. Based on years of canine nutritional research and our feeding experiences as the significant humans of six large dogs, we have concluded that a properly formulated home-prepared diet, based on a variety of whole foods with additional nutritional supplements, is the surest way to guarantee that your dog receives the nutrition s/he needs to develop and maintain a maximum level of health.

While dogs can thrive by eating the same foods as humans, they are inherently carnivorous. This means that their nutritional requirements differ from ours. For instance, dogs have a much greater need for protein and calcium than we do. They also have short digestive tracts and teeth that are designed to rip and tear food, rather than crush it as human teeth do. To accommodate these physical characteristics, the protein they consume must be easily digestible. Because domesticated dogs depend solely upon humans for their survival, it is incumbent upon us to understand their needs so we can do our best to ensure their health and happiness.

Feeding Our Dogs

FOR MUCH OF THEIR HISTORY, DOMESTICATED DOGS WERE fed a version of whatever their significant humans were eating, while wild dogs scavenged off the garbage from human settlements. As a result, the canine diet often consisted of vegetables, fruits, grains and table scraps — a combination that wasn't necessarily nourishing.

As previously noted, dogs need more calcium and protein than humans do. When grains and other plants are a dog's main sources of protein, essential amino acids are likely to be missing from the diet. Moreover, unless they are properly processed, plant proteins are likely to be difficult for dogs to digest. And a diet that comprises mainly table scraps is potentially high in fat and deficient in nutrients. A good diet should provide the full range and proper amounts of the essential nutrients that dogs need and be easily digestible to accommodate their short digestive tracts. When feeding your dog, a good rule to follow is, If you are not prepared to eat it yourself, don't feed it to your dog.

> ### ✚ DOC'S DOCTRINE
>
> The normal body temperature for an adult dog at rest at room temperature is 37.5–39.2°C or 99.5–102.6°F. The most accurate way to take a dog's temperature is to use either a rectal or an ear thermometer. A high temperature can indicate infection (bacterial or viral), inflammation or overheating. If your dog has a persistently high temperature, you should see your veterinarian.

The Matter of Table Scraps

ONE STARTING POINT FOR GETTING YOUR DOG ON THE road to good nutrition is understanding the difference between quality leftovers and table scraps. Most people have good-quality food left over from their meals, such as pieces of sirloin steak, roast beef, chicken or turkey. With any excess fat removed, these leftovers are fine to add to your dog's kibble or to use as the protein source in a properly formulated home-prepared diet. Leftover rice, pasta and safe vegetables (see "Foods that Are Known to Be Toxic to Dogs," page76) that are plainly cooked, with no butter or fatty sauces, can be used as carbohydrate sources in a home-prepared diet.

In addition to good-quality food, most people have bits of fatty or gristly meat and rich gravies or sauces left over from their meals. These table scraps are not nutritious, and we don't recommend feeding them to your dog.

Table Scraps as Dietary Enhancements

Today, dogs are not as likely to be fed a diet that consists entirely of table scraps as they were in the past. Instead, it is likely that table scraps are fed as embellishments to commercial dog food. Enhancing your dog's kibble with unhealthy table scraps is not a good idea. If you are adding table scraps to his/her diet, you are likely overfeeding your dog and predisposing him/her to obesity. By reducing the quantity of nutritionally balanced food and increasing the quantity of unhealthy table scraps, you are putting your dog at risk for nutritional deficiencies and possibly more-serious health problems. As previously noted, meat scraps are likely to be high in fat, and a diet that is too high in fat may contribute to gastrointestinal disorders, such as pancreatitis, a serious inflammation of the pancreas, which can be life-threatening.

> ### ✚ DOC'S DOCTRINE
>
> When dogs tuck their tails between their legs, they may be experiencing pain, discomfort or emotional distress.

Bandit

Recently, a three-year-old beagle named Bandit was brought to Grant's clinic with a history of vomiting, diarrhea, lethargy and a very sore stomach. Usually, Bandit was fed commercial dry food, but two days earlier, his family had treated him to a dinner of turkey meat with skin and gravy. Grant did some X-rays and blood work, which revealed that Bandit had pancreatitis. His problem was caused by his recent table-scraps feast. Fortunately, with treatment, he made a full recovery.

Processed Dog Food

WHILE COMMERCIAL DOG FOOD IS CONVENIENT AND often nutritious, it is not always an optimal diet for dogs. Even if you feed your dog the highest-quality commercially prepared dog food, his/her diet will still be lacking variety. Feeding your dog a variety of foods helps ensure that s/he is getting an adequate supply of vitamins, minerals and the other healthful components in food. Some animal nutritionists feel that you should change brands of commercially prepared food every couple of months to guard against your dog developing nutritional deficiencies. Eating a varied diet also helps to avoid potential toxicities; for example, liver may contain toxins and has high levels of vitamin A, which can be harmful when consumed in excess.

> ### ⊕ DOC'S DOCTRINE
>
> The average heart rate for dogs depends on their size. Smaller dogs have a resting heart rate of approximately 130 beats per minute, while large dogs have one of about 80 beats per minute. To take your dog's pulse, place your hand on the dog's chest or femoral artery (on the inside of the leg) to feel for the heart beats.

Recent developments in food science provide another reason why it makes sense to choose a home-prepared diet based on whole foods. Researchers are finding that eating whole foods seems to have health benefits that extend beyond providing good nutrition (see Whole Foods, page 20).

Though processed dog food that meets the standards of the Association of American Feed Control Officials (AAFCO) may be nutritionally sound, it can have other drawbacks. For instance, the quality of ingredients may be sacrificed to lower production costs. This means that ingredients not suitable for human consumption might be included in commercially prepared dog food. Moreover, food-processing procedures may destroy some nutrients. For instance, some vitamins and fatty acids become unstable when they are exposed to excessive heat or improperly stored. In addition, excessive heat can affect the digestibility of some types of protein.

In order to ensure a long shelf life and, therefore, be cost-effective, commercially prepared dog food usually includes preservatives and other additives. Some commercial dog foods contain synthetic preservatives, such as BHA, BHT and ethoxyquin. While preservatives are necessary to extend shelf life and prevent foods from becoming rancid, scientists don't fully understand the effect that many of these chemicals will have on the body over the long term.

Does Price Determine the Quality of the Food?

If you are feeding your dog commercially prepared food, don't let price determine your purchasing decision. The rule of thumb is, the lower the price the poorer the quality of ingredients. However, an expensive price tag does not necessarily mean that a food is better for your dog, and some high-quality mass-produced dog foods are very competitively priced due to economies of scale realized in the manufacturing and distribution processes. Make your purchasing decision based on the ingredient list and the label information, not the price.

Identifying Good-Quality Processed Foods

There are some very good processed dog foods on the market. When buying commercial dog food, read the label or product information carefully and look for the following:

- A statement that the food is nutritionally adequate to meet the maintenance or life-stage needs of your dog

- An animal-based protein source, such as beef, chicken, lamb and so on, as the predominant ingredient

- An expiry or processed-on date to guarantee freshness

- Natural preservatives, such as tocopherols (vitamin E) or vitamin C (Note: natural preservatives do not preserve food as long as synthetic preservatives do, especially after the bag is opened, so buy smaller quantities.)

- A digestibility factor of 80 to 90%

- Statement that the food has met AAFCO or similar criteria through humane feeding trials

- A recognizable or reputable brand-name manufacturer (look for the company's name, address and telephone number so you can contact them for product information — any manufacturer should be willing to answer questions about their products)

Commercial Foods and Home-Prepared Diets

Some pet-food companies have encouraged the myth that human food is not good for dogs. This is not surprising, since it is in their interest to promote the belief that commercially prepared products are the best choice for dogs. The problem is, some people are now afraid to feed their dogs fresh food because they believe it will be harmful.

Fortunately, many consumers are moving beyond this mind-set. They have begun to question the quality of the food they eat and are increasingly concerned about the safety of the food supply. As their interest in health, nutrition and food safety grows, it is natural that they broaden their interest and explore these issues with the long-term health of their companion animals in mind.

....

A New Breed of Commercial Dog Food

Today, the growing interest in home-prepared diets for dogs has spawned a new industry. People want to feed their dogs whole foods but still want the convenience of prepared meals. As a result, many companies are producing ready-made frozen meals for dogs that are much like frozen dinners for humans. Many of these products are based on raw-feeding theories (see Raw-Food Diets, page 25). Assess these prepared diets using the same approach you would for other commercially prepared food: most importantly, they should be nutritionally adequate.

• •

Whole Foods

IN THE WILD, DOGS SURVIVED ON whole foods. They consumed them fresh from the source and benefited from the full range of nutrients available in them. These foods were not altered by refining or processing and did not contain chemicals or additives, as many commercially processed dog foods do today.

Built around whole foods, a sensibly formulated home-prepared diet can provide the highest quality nutrition for your dog. It gives you the freedom to choose the ingredients you prefer, such as organically raised meats (free from potentially harmful therapeutic additives), whole grains and organically grown fruits and vegetables (free from pesticides). High-quality fresh or frozen whole foods also provide important nutrients and other compounds not found in processed food, which may offer additional health benefits.

Assessing Your Dog's Diet

After your dog has been on any diet for about a month, you should assess the most important reason for providing that food — the effect it has on his/her health. Consider the health of your dog's coat and skin and his/her energy level, weight and overall well-being. Have your veterinarian conduct wellness examinations and blood tests to monitor how well the diet is working for your dog.

For instance, researchers recently discovered components known as phytochemicals in foods. These natural compounds exist alongside nutrients and may have the potential to prevent many diseases, including cancer. The potential benefits of phytochemicals are derived from eating whole foods, as they appear to work in conjunction with other components of the food.

Know Good Health when You See It

A dog that is fed a well-balanced diet rich in beneficial nutrients shows many recognizable signs of good health. These include:

- Healthy coat that is soft and shiny and doesn't mat easily
- Little or no "doggie odor"
- Abundant energy
- Strong immune system, which keeps him/her healthy
- Brightness, a sparkle in his/her eyes and a sense that s/he is enjoying life
- Well-muscled body
- Well-formed stool that is not voluminous and is easily produced, with no straining

Problems Associated with Low-Quality Diets

Common problems associated with low-quality diets include:

- Skin odor
- Dull, greasy coat, usually accompanied by dandruff
- Susceptibility to generalized infections, such as ear infections that become chronic or skin infections caused by greasy, seborrheic skin
- Thin, undernourished appearance
- Low energy level
- Voluminous stool

Diet and Health: Personal Perspectives

NOTHING REINFORCES OUR BELIEFS ABOUT HOME-prepared diets more than our own experiences. In 1991, when he graduated from veterinary school, Grant had very limited knowledge of dogs' nutritional needs. The subject had not been taught in depth, and commercial pet-food manufacturers were the main source of information for veterinarians. It wasn't until he attended a course on complementary medicine, which featured nutrition as a major component, that he began to see the possibility of feeding dogs something other than commercial dog food.

Like many people, Grant made the transition to home-prepared dog food gradually. He began recommending that his clients feed their dogs higher-quality commercial foods, which contain better ingredients and natural preservatives (if not no preservatives). The turning point came when he used a natural, home-prepared diet to support a patient with a long-term debilitating disease.

> ### ⊕ DOC'S DOCTRINE
>
> The normal resting respiratory rate for adult dogs is approximately 22 breaths per minute. You can check the respiratory rate by watching and counting the up-and-down movement of the dog's rib cage for one minute. If you see increased respiratory effort, consult your veterinarian.

Sonny

Sonny, an 8-year-old male Chow Chow, had a devastating immune-system disease called *Pemphigus folliaceous*, which causes severe skin lesions on the face and paws. The main treatment for this disease is a long-term course of the corticosteroid prednisone. Sonny developed severe side effects from the drug, including liver and joint damage. As a result, Grant felt compelled to end Sonny's dependence on prednisone and the other medications he was receiving.

Grant consulted with a holistic veterinarian, who recommended a natural, home-prepared diet and herbal supplements. The results were amazing! Within weeks of beginning his new diet, Sonny had fewer skin lesions, and his coat became fuller and shinier. His quality of life improved dramatically: he was more alert, wanted to go on walks again and was more energetic throughout the day.

Otis

Grant was so impressed by the results he saw in Sonny that he began to do more research on home-prepared diets. He started to recommend natural, home-prepared food to other patients, often with the same results. He also saw the benefits with his own dog, Otis, then 14 years old. Otis, a 100-pound mixed-breed dog who was fed commercially prepared dry dog food, was going downhill quickly. His hind legs were becoming very weak, and he was losing weight. Also, his coat had become greasy, and he was constantly shedding. Grant decided to see if a natural, home-prepared diet would give his friend a much-needed boost.

Once again, the results were impressive. Within two weeks, the strength in his legs improved dramatically, as did his energy level. He could walk farther and rediscovered how much fun it was to chase a tennis ball. He gained back the weight he had lost, and his muscle tone improved. After a month on the diet, his coat became softer and shinier, and his greasy seborrhea disappeared. He started shedding seasonally instead of continuously.

The Five Dogs' Tale

> ### ✚ DOC'S DOCTRINE
>
> Dogs that chronically chew on or chase their tails may be suffering from various disorders, including flea-infestation, allergies, anal-gland disease or obsessive-compulsive behavior disorders. Your veterinarian can offer effective treatment options.

David and Jennifer are the significant humans of five large dogs — Harris, Zoee, Marley, Buffett and Dylan — and they have a similar story to tell. All of the dogs had been rescued from the local animal shelter after being identified as "unadoptable" because of various behavioral problems. Though they were traumatized by their unfortunate pasts, they soon adjusted to their new, loving environment, teaching their significant humans a valuable lesson in the power of not believing everything you hear — such as the word *unadoptable.*

Initially, David and Jennifer fed their dogs a premium dry commercial food and added small amounts of fresh foods, such as good-quality meats, rice and fresh vegetables, to make the kibble more palatable. But gradually they became concerned that while they were able to enjoy a wholesome, healthy diet with plenty of variety, their dogs ate the same processed food day in and day out. Questioning whether processed dog food was an optimum source of nutrition for their dogs, they began to explore home-prepared diets.

Switching their dogs to a home-prepared diet raised many questions. They wondered if they were doing it right, if they were missing important nutrients or if they might be feeding their dogs potentially harmful foods. But instead of answers, their research turned up a plethora of conflicting information on how home-prepared diets should be formulated and fed. Many of the sources seemed to be lacking scientific credibility.

Myths About Dogs and People Food

One prevalent myth is that feeding a dog freshly cooked meat will create a "taste for blood" and possibly incite the dog to kill other animals to satisfy that craving. While some dogs exhibit abnormal predatory behaviors, eating freshly cooked meat is likely not the cause. When dogs attack and kill prey, it is a behavioral, not a dietary, issue. Predation is a natural part of a dog's instincts. Predatory behavior is the basis of many canine behaviors that benefit humans, such as herding, tracking and hunting. Selective breeding and training has curbed the predatory instinct in most dogs, but it still finds an outlet in activities that are within the range of "normal" canine behavior — chasing cats, squirrels and bikes, for instance. Proper supervision, socialization and training can help keep such behavior under control.

One question we are often asked is, "Won't dogs become prone to begging at the table if they get accustomed to 'people food'?" This is a training, not a dietary, issue. If dogs are encouraged to eat in their own spaces and never fed from the table, they will, most likely, not beg for food from the table.

They raised their concerns with Grant, who had also been working with home-prepared diets. After some discussion, the three decided to pool their knowledge and research. Through further research, and justification through feeding trials with their own dogs, they concluded that the ideal diet should consist of a specific ratio of protein, fat and carbohydrates. They also concluded that vitamin-and-mineral supplements were necessary to ensure balance and achieve optimal nutrition. Eventually, they submitted their diet-formulation theory to a leading specialist in the field of canine nutrition, who gave them a positive evaluation.

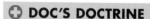

⊕ DOC'S DOCTRINE

Pack hierarchy is very important to dogs. Consistent reinforcement of your alpha (dominant) position through positive training, exercise and feeding practices is important to ensure the stability of the pack or family unit.

Raw-Food Diets

BELIEVE IT OR NOT, HOW A WHOLE-FOOD DIET SHOULD BE fed is a contentious issue in the dog world. The issue is whether food should be raw or cooked. While raw-food proponents make a good argument, we think the decision to feed a dog a raw-food diet should be approached very cautiously.

Advocates of the BARF (Biologically Appropriate Raw Food or Bones and Raw Food) diet and other raw-food diets fundamentally believe that because dogs originally ate raw food, they should still get their nutrients from fresh, raw foods. The theory is that the enzymes and nutrients a dog needs to remain healthy can be lost in the cooking process. Raw-food advocates report many health benefits from their diets, such as better breath and coat, longer life span and even cures for some diseases.

Although the ingredients vary with the diet, raw-food diets usually consist of raw, meaty bones; raw muscle meat (often from chicken); and raw organ meat — or any locally available meat, including beef, pork, poultry, rabbit or sheep. Raw fish, eggs (with shells), vegetables and ripe fruit; yogurt; cottage cheese; various yeasts; kelp (seaweed); and other natural supplements are also recommended. Depending on the diet, the quantity of grain included can range from very little to none at all.

....

A Potential for Contamination

On the other side of the raw-food debate are those who argue that the potential risks associated with feeding a dog a diet of raw meat and bones far outweigh the possible benefits. For starters, there is a very high potential for raw meat to be contaminated with salmonella and E. coli bacteria. These can pose a serious health threat not only to dogs but also to their significant humans, particularly young children, elderly family members and people with compromised immune systems. All it may take to get infected is a lick on the face from the dog or contact with the contaminated food bowl.

Some raw-food advocates argue that organically raised meat is less likely to be contaminated by bacteria and therefore safer to feed to a dog. This view, however, is not entirely correct. While the potential health risks associated with chemical and therapeutic additives used in standard farming practices are eliminated, organically raised meat may be more at risk for bacterial and parasitic contamination precisely because it lacks these additives. There are many reasons why organic meat may be preferable, but it must be thoroughly cooked in order to kill potentially harmful bacteria.

Many testimonials allege that dogs fed raw-food diets have experienced dramatic improvements in their health. Whether the meat is raw or cooked is likely secondary to the introduction of whole foods — a welcome change if the dog was previously fed low-quality commercially prepared food. However, there are many anecdotal examples of dogs becoming sick on raw-meat diets. Some cases have even resulted in death. One breeder we know lost two whippet puppies after they were fed raw chicken infected with salmonella. We asked a toxicologist and a researcher in the field of companion-animal nutrition for their opinions on raw-meat diets, and neither

> ### ✚ DOC'S DOCTRINE
>
> Do you want your female dog to live longer? Have her spayed before her first heat. This decreases her risk of mammary cancer to almost zero.

advocates the practice. Both felt that there is too much potential for contamination and that the danger this poses to the dog is too great. While some dogs seem to do well on raw-meat diets, we feel that the risk of bacterial infection outweighs any potential benefits. As a result, we cannot recommend feeding your dog a raw-meat diet. (For further reading on raw-food diets, see Resources, page 208.)

see Resources, page 208.

Other Potential Risks

Another concern is that some raw foods contain components that may interfere with the body's ability to use certain essential nutrients. When these foods are cooked, the harmful components are deactivated or destroyed, making them safer to consume. For instance, raw egg whites contain a protein called avidin, which binds up biotin (one of the B vitamins) so that the body is unable to use it. Therefore, including too many raw eggs in a diet can cause a biotin deficiency. Cooking the eggs deactivates the avidin.

Some types of raw fish contain a compound called thiaminase, which can interfere with the utilization of thiamin, one of the B vitamins. Cooking inactivates this compound, too. Raw salmon from the West Coast of North America presents an even more serious problem, as it may harbor a parasite that causes a canine condition known as salmon poisoning disease. This disease has symptoms that are similar to those of distemper or parvovirus and can be fatal if left untreated. Cooking the salmon kills this parasite.

Bones as Raw Food

Advocates of raw-food diets also recommend feeding bones to dogs to supply calcium. While a raw bone is less likely than a cooked bone to splinter and lodge in a dog's digestive tract, the risk is still present. Some raw-food proponents suggest that grinding bones into a powder before feeding them to a dog eliminates this danger. However, it is still possible for dangerous splinters to be present if the bones have been less-than-thoroughly ground.

. . . .

Canine Vegetarians?

SOME PROPERLY BALANCED, SO-CALLED VEGETARIAN DIETS can supply the nutrients dogs need to survive. For instance, there are people who exclude red meat from their diets but consume poultry and fish and call themselves vegetarians. Lacto-ovo vegetarians don't eat meat, poultry or fish but consume milk, milk products and eggs. Either of these two types of vegetarianism, when fed in a balanced formulation along with appropriate dietary supplementation, can be suitable for a dog.

The strictest vegetarians, known as vegans, don't eat or use any animal products whatsoever. As a result, vegans must meet their protein requirements by eating a variety of plant sources. Because plants lack a number of essential amino acids, unlike animal sources of protein, they are not complete and need to be judiciously combined in order to supply complete proteins.

Because plant sources of protein are incomplete, they are not optimal sources of protein for dogs. They are also more difficult for dogs to digest. As previously noted, dogs have short digestive tracts, which means they need easily digestible sources of protein. Moreover, their teeth, which are designed for eating meat, are not effective at crushing plant matter. These factors make it difficult for a dog on a vegan diet to get adequate levels of protein. Another concern is that some food plants — such as many members of the legume family and certain vegetables and fruits, including grapes, onions, avocados and broccoli — contain antinutritional factors or naturally occurring toxins that can be harmful to dogs. This limits the ingredients that can be used in a vegan

> ## ✚ DOC'S DOCTRINE
>
> Do you want your male dog to live longer? Neutering a male puppy before puberty (8 to 10 months of age) can help to prevent inappropriate male behaviors. More importantly, neutering an adult male dog before he is 6 years old prevents prostatic enlargement and infection, and anal-muscle diseases.

The Canine Diet

diet, which may lead to deficiencies due to insufficient variety. Another issue is vitamin B12, which is a necessary nutrient for dogs. Suitable amounts of this vitamin occur naturally only in animal sources. Because a vegan diet elevates your dog's risk of developing nutritional deficiencies, we cannot recommend it as a suitable option.

No Doggie Vegans

An exclusively plant-based diet is not suitable for dogs because:

- Plants do not contain complete proteins
- Plants are difficult for dogs to digest
- Some food plants can be toxic to dogs
- Plants are not a source of vitamin B12, which dogs need
- Dogs belong to the carnivore (meat-eating) group

Fasting

FASTING IS THE PRACTICE OF ABSTAINING FROM FOOD BUT not water for a period of time. Humans fast for spiritual and religious reasons, as well as for alleged health benefits. Fasting is thought to allow the body to rid itself of accumulated toxins and give the organs an opportunity to rest. It is also believed that fasting allows a body in ill health to repair itself more efficiently, as it does not have to use energy to digest food.

The practice of forcing dogs to fast for potential health benefits has been gaining in popularity. However, in our opinions, there are no circumstances that justify withholding food from a healthy dog. Proponents of fasting believe that because dogs' ancestors probably ate on irregular schedules, periodic fasting reflects a more natural and healthier feeding pattern. Although dogs living in the wild likely did fast, it was probably because they couldn't find anything to eat, not because they chose to.

There are some circumstances in which it is appropriate to fast a sick dog. However, this should only be undertaken under the supervision of a veterinarian and never for longer than 24 hours. The most common reason is to resolve large-bowel diarrhea. Restricting food intake gives the bowel a chance to heal before more food is presented. The fast is recommended for a 24-hour period and always includes plenty of fresh water. At that point, the dog is fed a bland diet until symptoms disappear.

Dogs Like Routine

One problem with fasting for nontherapeutic reasons is that some dogs may find it psychologically distressing. Stable routines are very important to dogs and they depend on them for their mental well-being. This is particularly true for those with certain anxiety-based problems. The psychological trauma a dog may experience when food is withheld far outweighs any potential benefits, should they exist.

Dogs and Diet-Related Health Problems

Obesity

Obesity, which is defined as having excess body fat, is a common disorder in companion animals. Quantity of food consumed, activity level and diet formulation can all play roles in obesity. A diet that is too high in fat and carbohydrates will provide more calories than a dog can use. The body stores this excess energy as fat.

Obesity is a dangerous condition. In addition to having a negative effect on a dog's overall health and life span, it can aggravate musculoskeletal diseases, such as arthritis (joint disease) in the hips, knees or elbows. It can also lead to other

The Canine Diet

health problems, including diabetes and respiratory ailments. Obesity can also make a dog more susceptible to spinal diseases, such as disc prolapse.

Some Dogs Are More Prone to Obesity

Before she was fed a home-prepared diet, David and Jennifer's dog Zoee had a weight problem. After adopting Zoee from the animal shelter, they discovered that she had a broken leg that had never been treated. By the time she came to live with them, Zoee had developed arthritis in that leg, which made it difficult for her to manage anything but moderate exercise. As a result, she put on weight and looked so large that David and Jennifer found themselves making excuses for her, such as, "She isn't fat; she's fluffy." Low-fat and calorie-reduced foods didn't help. In fact, Zoee's weight didn't go down to a healthy level until they began feeding her a home-prepared diet. Once they developed a sense of the ingredients that worked best for her and took control of the calories she was fed, David and Jennifer watched Zoee become her truly elegant self. Now they can say in all sincerity, "She isn't fat; she's fluffy."

➕ DOC'S DOCTRINE

Is your dog scooting or dragging his/her hind end along the ground? This behavior is usually caused by full or infected anal glands or, rarely, by intestinal parasites. Infected anal glands can rupture, causing severe pain requiring surgical repair. See your veterinarian for appropriate treatments.

The Causes of Obesity

Zoee's handicap was a contributing factor to her weight problem. However, there are many other reasons why dogs become obese: body type, lifestyle and certain health conditions can predispose them to obesity. A dog with a short-legged, stocky body type is more likely to become obese than a long-legged, slim dog. Not receiving enough exercise and being fed excessive amounts are lifestyle factors that can make a dog obese. And health conditions such as hypothyroidism can also predispose a dog to obesity. To avoid the health problems caused by excess weight, it is important to monitor your dog's weight on a regular basis.

➕ DOC'S DOCTRINE

Has your dog started drinking more water than normal? Overdrinking is a sign of internal disease, including metabolic diseases such as diabetes, Cushing's disease and kidney disease. It is important to consult with your veterinarian for diagnosis and treatment.

and take the appropriate steps to guard against obesity through suitable diet and exercise (see Checking Weight, page 66, for an easy way to check your dog's weight without a scale).

The Immune System

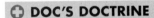
The immune system is a complicated mechanism that relies heavily on dietary nutrients to function properly. Vitamins, minerals, proteins, fats, carbohydrates and water are integral to its health, and the quality and quantity of these components also influence its performance. This link is clinically obvious: dogs that are well cared for and well nourished have fewer diseases.

If a dog consumes a diet deficient in any of the essential nutrients, his/her immune system may not function properly. Dogs are constantly exposed to bacteria, viruses and allergens. To neutralize these invaders, their immune systems must be able to adapt quickly. Poor nutrition can cause your dog's immune system to become overactive, which may result in devastating imbalances in his/her level of red blood cells, or it may cause it to be underactive, reducing the body's ability to fight infection. This often results in greater susceptibility to generalized infections or chronic ear, skin and bladder infections. A well-nourished body is able to channel optimal amounts of nutrients to the immune system so it can function at its highest level.

> "In clinical practice, we definitely see a link between good nutrition and a dog's ability to fight infection and control chronic disease."
> — Dr. Grant Nixon

Jess

One of Grant's patients, an older black Lab named Jess, had a long struggle with chronic, intermittent pneumonia. Although the illness responded to antibiotics, three to four weeks after the drugs were finished the symptoms invariably returned. Grant recommended a home-prepared diet. Eight weeks later, when she returned for a checkup, Jess was symptom-free. It was exciting to see such a clear link between diet and better health.

Greasy Coat, Dandruff and Doggie Odor

If your dog has a greasy coat or dandruff, it's because the oil-secreting glands in the skin are inflamed and oversecreting oil. The oil accumulates in the coat and binds to microscopic skin flakes, causing the clumps that we recognize as dandruff. Too much oil in the coat causes the unpleasant smell that many dogs emit. The amount and types of fat present in the diet have a direct impact on these problems. To promote skin and coat health, dogs need the right amount of essential fatty acids. If their diets are deficient in essential fatty acids, skin and coat problems will result.

Chronic Ear Infections

If a dog is undernourished, the first areas to suffer are nonvital ones, such as the skin and external ear canal. S/he may have excessive ear-wax secretions, which make him/her more prone to infection. Water in the ear, metabolic disease and poor nutrition can also compromise the defense system of the ear. As a result, bacteria or yeast that normally live inside the ear canal in small numbers can proliferate and cause painful infections. Once an infection is established, the undernourished immune system will be unable to eradicate it.

> **✚ DOC'S DOCTRINE**
>
> Does your dog shake his/her head a lot? This can indicate an ear infection. Chronic ear infections can cause severe pain and shorten your dog's life span. Ears that smell bad or sour are a clear sign of an ongoing ear infection that is caused by bacteria, yeast or mites. Consult your veterinarian for a complete treatment protocol.

In clinical practice, Grant sees many dogs with chronic ear infections and greasy, dull coats. He has learned that proper medical treatment combined with improved nutrition, such as from a home-prepared diet, not only treats the disease but also controls recurrence.

Gastrointestinal Problems

While there are obvious connections between diet and gastrointestinal upsets such as indigestion and gas, diet can also be a factor in serious gastrointestinal diseases, including pancreatitis (inflammation of the pancreas, often associated with a high-fat diet), inflammatory bowel disease (a broad group of diseases involving the stomach, small intestine or colon) and colitis (large-bowel irritation usually caused by dietary indiscretions).

Diet Can Help

One significant benefit of a home-prepared diet is your ability to tailor the diet to meet your dog's individual needs. David and Jennifer's dog Marley is a case in point. When Marley was eating premium commercial dog food, he had gastrointestinal problems: uncomfortable gas and chronically loose or runny stools. David and Jennifer tried a number of methods to alleviate these problems, such as switching foods, dispensing antacids and adding digestive enzymes and dietary supplements to Marley's diet, all to no avail.

> ✚ **DOC'S DOCTRINE**
>
> Your dog is an important family member that you want to keep safe. Permanent identification can be an invaluable asset in finding a lost dog. Options include a microchip implanted under the skin or a tattoo in the ear or on the flank.

Within days of feeding Marley a home-prepared diet, they noticed results: his gas problem was completely alleviated, and his stools firmed up. Just like that! No more gas. No more groans. No more sighs. In addition, Marley seemed to have a new lease on life. He was more playful with the other dogs in the yard. On family hikes, he ran or trotted instead of plodding along. After he had been on the home-prepared diet for about three weeks, they noticed dramatic changes in his coat. It was softer, shinier and did not feel greasy. Marley continues to be gas-free and very healthy.

> ✚ **DOC'S DOCTRINE**
>
> Rolling in smelly things like manure, dead animals or garbage is a normal behavior for a dog. Some experts theorize that this is atavistic behavior from the days when dogs tried to cover their scent for hunting.

More Diet-Related Diseases

Other diseases in which diet can be a factor are various cancers, immune-mediated diseases, skeletal diseases, infectious diseases and dental diseases.

Behavioral Problems

The correlation between behavior and diet seems logical; for instance, common sense suggests that a sedentary dog should not be fed a nutrient-dense diet designed for working dogs, such as police, sled or hunting dogs. Obesity or hyperactivity would be logical results. Similarly, an active dog that does not receive the extra nutrients s/he needs to maintain an appropriate amount of energy will be undernourished. This could lead to inappropriate behaviors, such as scavenging garbage, stealing food, coprophagy (eating feces) or anxiety-driven behavioral disorders. A diet for any dog should provide the proper number of calories and amounts of nutrients that correspond to his/her weight and lifestyle.

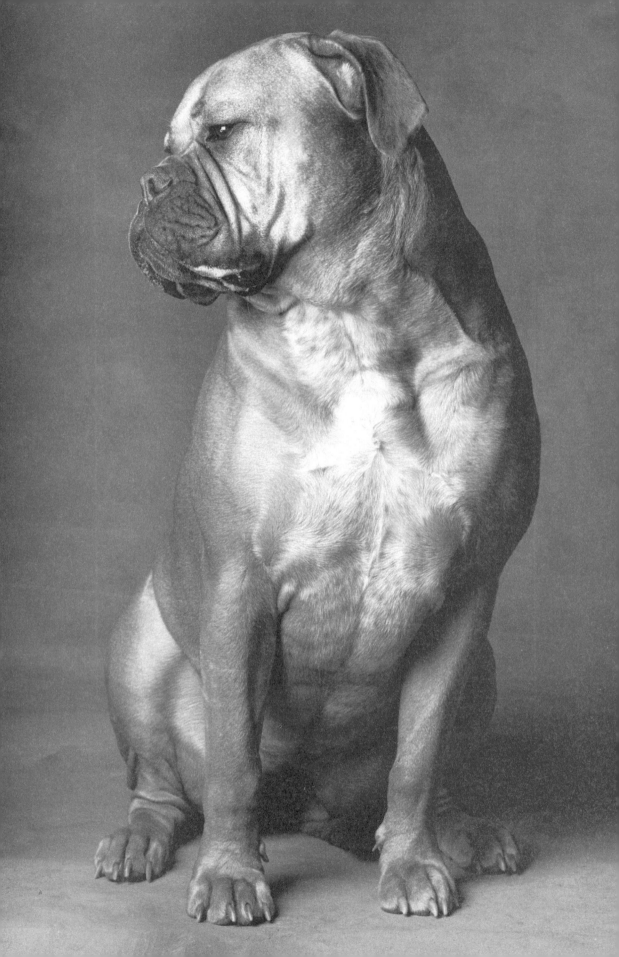

Better Food for Dogs

GEORGIA — 20-MONTH-OLD BULLMASTIFF

Diet Formulation: A Sensible Approach

A DOG'S MEAL NEEDS TO BE MORE THAN JUST A COMBInation of tasty ingredients. His/her diet must be formulated based on a thorough understanding of canine nutritional needs. This includes knowing what foods supply the nutrients that are essential for dogs, what additional supplements are needed and what quantity of food and supplements will provide enough energy to sustain good health and enable your dog to be as active as s/he needs to be.

In formulating our diet, we have used information provided by the National Research Council (NRC), the United States Department of Agriculture (USDA), Health Canada and the Association of American Feed Control Officials (AAFCO), among other sources.

Both the NRC and the AAFCO have set standards for canine nutritional requirements, and this information is available through various publications (for further reading, see Resources, page 209). The USDA and Health Canada have provided nutrient information on common foods, which is also available (see Resources, page 209).

Our recipes have been created based on diet-formulation principles that, in our opinions, take a sensible approach to feeding your dog a home-prepared diet. The ratio of fats,

---

Monitor the Diet

When feeding your dog this or any other diet, including commercially prepared dog food, we recommend working with your veterinarian to monitor its suitability. No one diet formulation can meet every dog's individual needs perfectly. Chapter 3 provides a fuller description of the various tools we recommend for assessing the diet's efficacy on an ongoing basis.

---

protein and carbohydrates conforms to nutritional guidelines. Nutritional supplements are added to ensure that required nutrient levels are achieved. Our diet-formulation theory has received a positive evaluation from specialists in the field of canine nutrition and has been studied further in feeding trials with our own dogs. Excellent results in wellness testing and blood work on our dogs confirm its efficacy.

Make It Tasty

The purpose of a good diet is to supply your dog with optimal nutrition to meet his/her energy requirements and support good health. However, no matter how nutritionally sound any diet is, if your dog doesn't like the taste of what you put in his bowl and refuses to eat, the diet has failed.

Happy Birthday, Otis

Fortunately, reluctance to eat isn't a problem with Grant's dog, Otis — he loves his home-cooked food. And his friends are discovering the joys of home cooking, as well. When Otis turned 100 in equivalent people years, his family celebrated by making him a meat-loaf "cake," with cooked rib bones as candles, and invited his friends Natuck and Casey to a birthday party. After singing "Happy Birthday," they removed the bones and gave the dogs a piece of "cake." Otis launched into eating with his usual gusto, but Natuck and Casey, unaccustomed to home-cooked food, went wild with delight. Casey decided he needed a second piece and shouldered old-timer Otis out of the way to grab what was left of his. Natuck zeroed in on the table and helped herself to the cake that remained in the pan. Watching Natuck and Casey show such enthusiasm for food was a real eye-opener for their significant humans, who have since taken a more active interest in what they feed their dogs.

> ### ✚ DOC'S DOCTRINE
> Carsickness is very common in dogs and can be caused by the motion of the car or by anxiety. You can acclimatize your dog to the car by just sitting in it and not going anywhere. Then build up to short rides to help your dog overcome this problem. Do not feed a dog that is prone to carsickness within four hours of a planned car ride.

The Joys of Home Cooking

One advantage of home-prepared diets is that they offer the freedom to choose the ingredients that your dog eats. They allow you to discover the foods that your best friend enjoys and benefits from. They also strengthen the bond between you and your dog by introducing elements of pleasure and fun into mealtime. All our Basic Recipes include variations, which suggest a variety of ingredients that can be substituted for those in the master recipe. We have also included a list of common ingredients and substitutions for them (see Substituting Ingredients, page 87).

Varying the ingredients in your dog's diet does more than just whet his/her appetite by banishing the not-the-same-old-thing-again blahs; it helps ensure that s/he gets the full range of available nutrients and guards against toxicity, which may result from eating too much of certain foods. You can even add flavor enhancers, such as herbs and spices, in small amounts — just be sure they won't cause adverse reactions (see Foods that Are Known to be Toxic to Dogs, page 76).

Kilocalories (kcal)

The energy value that a food supplies is measured in a large calorie unit called a kilocalorie (kcal). A small calorie is the amount of energy that it takes to raise the temperature of one gram of water by 1°C. As this small unit of measurement is too difficult to use to express food energy, it is expressed as kcal (1,000 times larger than a small calorie). When a calorie is expressed as Calorie (with a capital C), it is usually referring to a kcal.

> ### Seal of Approval
> All of the recipes in this book have met with the enthusiastic approval of all of our dogs — even Buffett, who is a very finicky eater!

· ·

The Diet Formula

WE HAVE BASED ALL OUR RECIPES ON the following formula. This diet is intended for use by adult dogs that have no special dietary needs due to state of health or environment (climate) and that are not pregnant, lactating or working dogs — such as police dogs.

In addition to the proper levels of essential nutrients, dogs should always have an adequate supply of fresh, clean water.

Always feed dogs twice a day, as feeding smaller meals more often improves digestibility.

> ### ✚ DOC'S DOCTRINE
> If you are a smoker, here is a good reason to quit: secondhand smoke can be very harmful to your dog. It can increase his/her risk of cancer and allergic disease.

The Essential Nutrients

The macronutrients a dog needs to thrive should be provided in the following ratio:

- 40% of total kcal from a protein source
- 45% of total kcal from carbohydrate sources (35% cooked grains plus 10% vegetable and/or fruit)
- 15% of total kcal from a supplemental fat (oil) source

In addition, the following micronutrients should be added:

- sodium chloride (table salt) and/or potassium chloride (salt substitute), depending upon the ingredients used in the meal
- bonemeal and a multivitamin-and-mineral supplement

Nutrient Sources
for Your Dog

Proteins

Proteins provide the building materials (amino acids) that are necessary for growth, maintenance and repair of tissues, organs, blood and hair. They are essential to many vital functions and are used by the body as a source of energy.

Proteins are made up of essential and nonessential amino acids. Dogs can produce nonessential amino acids through normal bodily functions. However, they cannot meet their requirements for essential amino acids on their own; their diet must supply them.

If, over time, a dog doesn't get enough protein, or the protein is deficient in essential amino acids, serious consequences may result. These include anorexia, slowed growth, greater susceptibility to infection, depression, hypoproteinemia (low protein levels in the blood), emaciation and even death.

Sources of Protein

The best sources of protein for dogs are:

- Meat
- Poultry
- Fish
- Eggs
- Organ meat
- Some dairy products, such as cottage cheese

All Proteins Aren't Equal

Most foods contain some protein. The problem is, all proteins aren't equal. High-quality proteins should be easily digestible, as dogs have short digestive tracts. Proteins should also be complete, meaning that they should contain all the essential amino acids. Most animal proteins — which are found in meat, fish, poultry, eggs and some dairy products — meet these fundamental criteria.

Proteins from animal sources are preferable for dogs, as they are complete proteins that dogs can easily digest. Plant-based proteins are incomplete, as they lack a number of amino acids. In order to create a complete protein, a plant-based protein must be combined with a carbohydrate, such as brown rice, to supply the complete range of amino acids. Another concern with feeding plant-based proteins is that they are difficult for dogs to digest unless they are properly processed. As a result, we do not feel that plant-based foods are a good source of protein for dogs.

Carbohydrates

Carbohydrates have many uses in the body. When they are broken down by the digestive system and converted to glucose (the major sugar in the blood that is used for energy), they supply fuel for activity. They also supply fiber, which aids gastrointestinal function.

Sources of Carbohydrates

Carbohydrate sources suitable for a dog's diet include:

- Cooked whole grains, such as brown rice, oatmeal and barley
- Whole wheat flour products, including whole-grain breads and pastas
- Potatoes
- Vegetables and fruits that are safe for dogs to consume (see Foods that Are Known to Be Toxic to Dogs, page 76)

Whether carbohydrates should be included in a dog's diet has been the subject of much debate, due to the dog's ancestry as a carnivore. Because, even in the wild, carnivores consume carbohydrates (often from the intestinal tracts of their prey), it is generally agreed that dogs need some carbohydrates. It's the amount of carbohydrates required to maintain health that is the subject of debate. Paradoxically, carbohydrates are often a major source of energy in commercial dog foods. However, recent studies show that dogs do need carbohydrates and benefit from their inclusion in their diets.

✚ DOC'S DOCTRINE

Do you rely on your dog's wet nose to indicate good health? A change in the condition of the nose (wet to dry or dry to wet) is a better indicator of internal disease.

Feeding Carbohydrates

When including carbohydrates in your dog's diet, keep the following points in mind.

- Too many carbohydrates can cause gas, diarrhea or weight gain.

- Grains must be cooked so your dog can digest them properly.

- Brown rice is the best cooked grain, as it is rich in nutrients and easily digestible.

- If a vegetable needs to be cooked before you can eat it, you will need to cook it for your dog.

- Puree raw fruits and vegetables so your dog will be able to digest them properly.

- Leave the skin on most fruits and vegetables. Use common sense: if you need to peel it for yourself, peel it for your dog. Discard any pits or seeds, as they may be toxic or cause your dog to choke.

- If you are introducing new vegetables or fruits into your dog's diet, observe his/her reactions carefully, because some dogs have difficulty tolerating certain foods (see Foods that Are Known to Be Toxic to Dogs, page 76).

Mix Well for Optimum Health

We recommend feeding your dog a variety of foods to ensure that his/her nutritional needs are met. Varying the sources of protein and carbohydrates in your dog's diet — for instance, feeding Beef and Rice with one vegetable-and-fruit mix early in the week, then Chicken and Potatoes and a different vegetable-and-fruit mix later in the week — broadens the range of nutrients your dog receives and helps achieve nutrient balance. (If your dog has a problem tolerating a food change within a week, then space any changes out over a slightly longer period of time.) Variety also helps guard against toxicity from vitamin or mineral excesses and overexposure to naturally occurring toxins that may be present in some foods. As the nutrient content of foods varies from place to place, season to season and product to product, it also helps to ensure that nutritional deficiencies relating to the food supply are less likely to occur.

Fats

Fats are a highly concentrated form of food energy. They supply essential fatty acids and serve as carriers for the fat-soluble vitamins: A, D, E and K. Fat deposits in the body protect and stabilize various internal organs and insulate the body. Fats also add flavor to food, making mealtime a more pleasurable experience for your dog.

Keeping a close eye on the quantity of fat in your dog's diet is important, because fat contains twice as many calories as protein or carbohydrates. Protein and carbohydrates supply approximately 4.5 kcal per gram, while fats provide approximately 9 kcal per gram. If too many calories come from fat, s/he may not get enough essential nutrients from other protein or carbohydrate food sources. This can lead to serious nutritional deficiencies over time. Moreover, too much fat can lead to serious health problems, such as obesity and pancreatitis.

Essential Fatty Acids

Fats supply essential fatty acids, which play many important roles in the body. Dogs have a recognized requirement for linoleic acid, the main fatty acid in a category of polyunsaturated fatty acids (PUFAs) known as omega-6. Omega-6 fatty acids play an important role in skin and coat health, tissue repair, immune-system response and reproductive function. Dogs must get linoleic acid in their diets because it can not be manufactured by the body. If your dog's diet is deficient in essential fatty acids, s/he may be more susceptible to skin disorders, coat problems and infection. Vegetable oils such as safflower or canola are good sources of linoleic acid. Some meats — especially the dark meat, fat and skin of chicken — are also good sources of linoleic acid. In order to control fat intake and ensure a consistent supply of linoleic acid, we use lean meats in all our recipes, then we add canola oil. When adding an oil supplement such as this to your dog's diet, introduce it gradually, as diarrhea may result if it is introduced too quickly.

Omega-3s

Alpha-linolenic acid is the head of a category of PUFAs known as omega-3. Although omega-3 fatty acids are not considered essential to dogs, they have been shown to have health benefits when added to the diet in moderate amounts. One benefit is that omega-3s can aid in the treatment of skin disease and arthritis by regulating the body's inflammatory and immune responses. Fatty fish, such as salmon, is a rich source of omega-3 fatty acids and can, on occasion, serve as an alternate source of protein in your dog's diet.

While some omega-3s can be beneficial to include in the diet, oversupplementation of omega-3s should be avoided, as it may depress the immune system. This can lead to a greater risk of infection, especially in dogs whose immune systems have been compromised. Giving your dog omega-3 fatty acid supplements should only be undertaken with the guidance of your veterinarian.

Water

Water is the most essential of all the dietary components that humans and dogs need to survive. Dogs can survive for an extended period of time without food but will die very quickly without water. Water needs to be replenished on a regular basis, as it is lost quite quickly through urination, breathing and other physiological processes. Water is usually obtained through drinking, but food also helps supply water to the body.

A dog should have constant access to clean, fresh water. This is especially important when the climate is hot. Dogs are poor thermoregulators, so they need to lose heat through the mouth and respiratory tract. Therefore, dogs cool themselves by panting, not by sweating. In the heat, dogs pant heavily, making them more prone to dehydration. If a dog is dehydrated, the efficiency of heat loss through panting will decrease.

Adding Necessary Supplements

IN THEORY, THE RIGHT COMBINATION and quantity of food from all the food groups should provide an adequate supply of nutrients. However, this balance can be difficult to achieve, as the nutritional quality of foods varies dramatically and can be affected by a diverse range of factors, from cooking techniques to the season in which the food was harvested. In our opinions, supplementing home-prepared diets with additional vitamins and minerals is

> ### Ask Your Pharmacist
> Our search for a multivitamin-and-mineral supplement to meet the needs of our large dogs was a challenge as we couldn't find a single capsule that provided the full range of essential vitamins and minerals. We found a product that met most of their daily requirements (with 2 capsules), although the levels of vitamin B12, iodine and choline were not sufficient. We took our chosen supplement to our local pharmacist, who was very helpful in directing us toward additional supplements that would provide sufficient levels of the missing nutrients without creating toxic levels of those which might be a concern (see Toxicity Levels of Vitamins and Minerals, page 196). He also provided useful information on the quality of multivitamin-and-mineral supplements, which varies, particularly in the minerals. When buying mineral supplements, look for the chelated variety. They are more costly than most, but are much more readily absorbed by the body than oxides or sulfates.

necessary to ensure that your dog's nutrient requirements are met.

Multivitamin-and-Mineral Supplements

When choosing a multivitamin-and-mineral supplement, it is important to find one that is suitable for use with a home-prepared diet. Many of the multivitamin-and-mineral supplements on the market are not suitable for dogs eating home-prepared diets because they are too low in nutrients. Many are intended for use with commercial dog food, which already contains additional vitamins and minerals. Before feeding your dog a multivitamin-and-mineral supplement, use the charts in Chapter 7 to be sure it offers the appropriate levels of vitamins and minerals and check with your veterinarian to ensure that it offers a balanced formulation for your dog. Although there are some excellent supplements on the market that work well with a home-prepared diet, depending upon where your live, they may be difficult to find. A simple solution is to use a daily multivitamin-and-mineral supplement intended for humans. When purchasing such a supplement, use the charts in Chapter 7 and consult with your pharmacist to ensure that you are adding the proper supplementation without reaching toxic levels.

> **Tip**
>
> When adding a multivitamin-and-mineral supplement intended for humans to your dog's diet, be sure to read the ingredient list carefully. Some human multivitamin-and-mineral supplements may contain added nutraceuticals (see Beyond Nutrition pg 51). The safety of some of these products for use with dogs may not be known, so choose a multivitamin-and-mineral supplement that is free of these extra ingredients.

Bonemeal

Dogs have a greater need for calcium than humans do. When feeding a home-prepared diet, a daily calcium supplement is required — not only to help your dog meet his/her calcium requirements but also to ensure that the ratio of calcium to phosphorus is appropriate in the diet. This ratio is 1.2 to 1.4 parts calcium to one part phosphorus. Maintaining the proper calcium-to-phosphorus ratio is important, because if there is more phosphorus than calcium in the diet, there will be signs of calcium deficiency even when an adequate level of calcium is actually present.

Phosphorus levels in a dog's diet can be quite high because meat is high in phosphorus and low in calcium. In the wild, dogs met their calcium needs by eating bones, which are high in calcium and low in phosphorus. Adding bonemeal to a home-prepared diet provides your dog with a good source of calcium, while avoiding the dangers associated with feeding bones. However, the bonemeal must be human-grade to avoid the high levels of toxins, such as lead, that are present in garden-grade bonemeal. The phosphorus levels in the bone-meal also need to be taken into consideration. Look for bonemeal at pet-supply stores, health-food stores and some veterinary clinics and consult the relevant chart for your dog's weight in Chapter 7 to learn how much bonemeal you will need to add to your dog's diet.

....

Salts

Dogs, like humans, need sodium, chloride and potassium to protect against dehydration and aid in bodily functions. Although fresh foods contain sodium and potassium, they may not contain enough of these electrolytes to meet canine requirements.

Depending on the ingredients used, you may need to add sodium chloride (table salt) and potassium chloride (salt substitute) to a recipe. For instance, potatoes contain relatively large amounts of potassium. If the quantity of potatoes is sufficient in a recipe, supplemental potassium is not required. Similarly, if processed human food products that contain high levels of sodium are called for, additional sodium may not be necessary.

> ### Iodine and Salt
> Iodized salt is a major source of iodine (an essential nutrient) in the recipes contained in this book. Even so, the multivitamin-and-mineral supplement should meet or get fairly close to a dog's minimum requirements for iodine, as shown in the charts in Chapter 7.

The amount of salt required also varies with the size of the dog. Too much salt can be detrimental to a dog's health, just as it can be to a human's. Add salt carefully, in accordance with the recipe instructions.

Vitamins

Vitamins are essential nutrients found in plant and animal food sources. They promote and regulate various physiological processes and protect the body from certain illnesses or conditions. Ideally, dogs should get most of their vitamins from food. Unlike humans, dogs can manufacture their own vitamin C.

Vitamins are divided into two groups: fat-soluble and water-soluble. The fat-soluble vitamins A, D, E and K are stored in the tissues and can build up and become toxic. Take care to ensure that your dog does not receive an excessive dose of any of these vitamins.

Macro- and Micronutrients

The vitamins and minerals that need to be added to your dog's diet are known as micronutrients. One of their many functions is to help the body utilize the macronutrients — protein, carbohydrates and fat — that are found in food. Micronutrients, in the form of supplements, are an essential component of a home-prepared diet. However, dogs, like people, can not live on supplements alone. The purpose of a home-prepared diet is to provide your dog with the proper ratio of macronutrients found in good-quality, highly digestible whole foods. Moreover, as discussed earlier (see Whole Foods page 20), in addition to nutrients, whole foods contain other compounds that may offer additional health benefits. It is the combination of good-quality, highly digestible ingredients and nutritional supplements that provides your dog with the optimal nutrition offered by a home-prepared diet.

A Fine Balance

The body uses very small amounts of vitamins and minerals, but prolonged deficiencies or excesses of some vitamins and minerals can have detrimental health effects, including, in extreme situations, death. This is why it is important to vary the ingredients in your dog's diet and to ensure that his/her food is properly supplemented.

The water-soluble vitamins are the B-complex vitamins (thiamin, riboflavin, niacin, pantothenic acid, pyridoxine, cyanocobalamin, folic acid, biotin and choline) and vitamin C. These vitamins are not stored in the body and are lost through urination. As a result, they need to be provided on a regular basis. For more information on the essential vitamins, see the chart on pages 52 to 53.

Beyond Nutrition

Part of the growing trend toward better canine health through diet includes the use of dietary supplements or nutraceuticals. A nutraceutical is a food or ingredient that may offer health benefits that go beyond basic nutrition.

Dietary supplements that are gaining popularity for use in dogs to treat specific conditions include:

- Glucosamine, chondroitin sulfate, MSM (methyl-sulfonyl-methane) and yucca (to aid in joint health for management of arthritis)
- Vitamin C, vitamin E, beta-carotene and selenium (antioxidants that protect against free-radical damage)
- Omega-3 fatty acids (to aid in the treatment of skin disease)
- Probiotics (good bacteria that aid digestion)
- A multitude of herbal remedies to treat various illnesses

Although many dietary supplements have been shown to have a positive effect on health, others have not been tested for efficacy or safety. Before giving your dog any dietary supplement, check with your veterinarian.

The Essential Vitamins

Vitamin	Functions	Deficiencies	Sources
Vitamin A	important in the maintenance of skin, vision and mucous membranes; assists in growth, including bone and tooth formation; improves immunity	anorexia, skin diseases, eye problems (including night blindness), ataxia (loss of balance) and increased risk of infection	orange and yellow vegetables, such as carrots and sweet potatoes; dark green leafy vegetables; eggs; liver; fish; and whole-milk products
Vitamin B1 (Thiamin)	helps transform carbohydrates into energy; vital to nerve, stomach and heart functions	cardiac disease, convulsions, anorexia, weight loss and abnormal reflexes	whole grains, organ meat, meat, fish and nuts
Vitamin B2 (Riboflavin)	assists in cellular growth, energy production and metabolism of nutrients	dry, reddened skin; anemia; hind-limb weakness; and eye lesions	whole grains, organ meat, eggs, dairy products and green leafy vegetables
Vitamin B3 (Niacin)	required for metabolism of nutrients	reddening and ulceration of the mouth and tongue (black tongue disease)	meat, fish, poultry, liver, whole grains, brewer's yeast and peanuts
Vitamin B5 (Pantothenic Acid)	assists in metabolism of nutrients and steroid production	weakened immune system, depressed growth, hypoglycemia, anorexia, increased blood urea nitrogen, fatty liver and convulsions	organ meat, eggs, whole grains, milk, fish and poultry
Vitamin B6 (Pyridoxine)	assists in metabolism of nutrients	anemia, anorexia and convulsions	meat, fish, whole grains, liver, green leafy vegetables, bananas and brewer's yeast
Vitamin B12 (Cyanocobalamin)	metabolism of nutrients; integral in the synthesis and maintenance of DNA, red blood cells and nerves	pernicious anemia	organ meat, meat, fish, dairy products and eggs
Folic Acid	important in the synthesis of DNA and in the development of red blood cells in bone marrow	anorexia and anemia	organ meat, dark green leafy vegetables, whole grains and cooked beans

Vitamin	Functions	Deficiencies	Sources
Biotin	important in the metabolism of nutrients and maintenance of skin, hair and nails	skin and coat problems, including hair loss and dry skin	widespread in foods, including meat, egg yolks, peanuts and many fruits and vegetables
Choline	nerve function and enzyme production; essential for the transport of fat from the liver	fatty liver and low levels of albumen (a protein present in the blood)	eggs, fish and organ meat
Vitamin C	antioxidant; assists in the formation of collagen and steroids; integral in immune-system function	no naturally occurring deficiencies in dogs, as they manufacture vitamin C; if deficiency occurs from other contributing factors, such as decreased liver function, symptoms may include retarded healing and increased susceptibility to disease	citrus fruits, melons, berries and tomatoes
Vitamin D	aids in the absorption of calcium; essential for proper growth and development of bones and teeth	bone-density loss in adult dogs and rickets in young dogs	fatty fish, dairy products, eggs and organ meat
Vitamin E	antioxidant; assists in circulation, reproduction and immune system function	impaired immunity, reproductive failure and eye problems	vegetable oils, green leafy vegetables, nuts, seeds and whole grains
Vitamin K	blood clotting	no simple deficiencies in dogs, as they can produce vitamin K in the intestines; if deficiency occurs from outside factors, such as ingestion of rat poison (specifically warfarin, a compound that interferes with blood clotting), symptoms include hemorrhage, anorexia and lethargy. Vitamin K administered orally can counteract warfarin poisoning	canola, safflower and olive oils; green leafy vegetables; soybeans; eggs; and liver

The Essential Minerals

Mineral	Functions	Deficiencies	Sources
MACROMINERALS			
Calcium (Ca)	essential for growth and maintenance of bones and teeth; aids in blood clotting and nerve function	loss of bone density, which can cause lameness, stiffness, chronic-spontaneous fractures, deviations of limbs and tooth loss	dairy products, dark green leafy vegetables, eggshells and bonemeal
Phosphorus (P)	related to calcium in bodily functions; aids in production of energy within cells	loss of bone density and fatigue	meat, eggs, dairy products, whole grains and bonemeal
Potassium (K)	essential in regulating body-fluid balance and heart and nervous system function	predisposition to dehydration, muscular paralysis and heart and kidney damage	lean meat, vegetables, fruits, whole grains and salt substitutes
Sodium (Na)	essential in regulating body-fluid balance	weakness, fatigue, inability to maintain body-fluid balance, decreased water consumption, loss of appetite, dry skin and hair loss	table salt. Sodium occurs naturally in foods but still needs to be added to a home-prepared diet, as the naturally occurring levels are usually inadequate. Note: processed foods, including cheese, bread products, some sauces and cured meats, can contain high levels of sodium
Chloride (Cl)	essential in regulating body-fluid balance; important component in the digestive juices of the stomach	weakness, fatigue, inability to maintain body-fluid balance, decreased water consumption, loss of appetite, dry skin, hair loss and impaired digestion	table salt
Magnesium (Mg)	important in energy production and maintenance of proper pH balance; component of muscle and bone	anorexia, weight loss, weakness and seizures	whole grains, dark green leafy vegetables, nuts and seafood

Mineral	Functions	Deficiencies	Sources
TRACE MINERALS			
Iron (Fe)	essential in hemoglobin and myoglobin production to prevent anemia; component of various enzymes	anemia	meat (especially red meat), organ meat, fish, poultry, green leafy vegetables, dried fruits and nuts
Copper (Cu)	essential, in conjunction with iron, in the prevention of anemia, hemoglobin production, enzymes and pigmentation of hair and skin	anemia	organ meat, seafood and nuts
Manganese (Mn)	important in energy production, cartilage growth, enzyme reactions and reproduction	reproductive failure (miscarriage), stiffness, joint problems and brittle bones	whole grains, green leafy vegetables, nuts and pineapples
Zinc (Zn)	important for skin health, protein and collagen formation, immune-system function and healing of wounds	skin disease; thick, scaly lesions on the extremities and abdomen, poor weight gain; and emaciation	meat and seafood
Iodine (I)	important in thyroid hormone production and energy regulation	goiter (enlargement of the thyroid gland), hair irregularities, drowsiness, cretinism (deformity and mental retardation) and apathy	iodized salt, seafood and kelp
Selenium (Se)	interaction with vitamin E, protection of cell membranes; immune function	weakness, muscular degeneration and anorexia	meat, fish, whole grains and Brazil nuts

Minerals

Like vitamins, minerals perform many valuable functions in the body. These include regulating body fluids, developing and maintaining bones and teeth, and keeping muscles and nerves functioning well.

Minerals are divided into two groups: macrominerals, which are found in greater concentrations in the body's tissues, and trace minerals. Though trace minerals are present in very small amounts, they are still essential.

Energy Requirements of the Adult Dog

DOGS' DAILY CALORIC REQUIREMENTS VARY. SIZE, WEIGHT, body type, breed, health status, age, coat type, environment (climate) and level of activity influence individual energy needs. This dictates that no one formula for calculating energy requirements is perfect for every dog.

Range of Daily Energy Requirements of Average Adult Dogs

Weight	Energy	Weight	Energy
5 lbs/2.3 kg	203–244 kcal	70 lbs/31.7 kg	1,471–1,766 kcal
10 lbs/4.5 kg	341–411 kcal	75 lbs/34.0 kg	1,549–1,859 kcal
15 lbs/6.8 kg	463–556 kcal	80 lbs/36.2 kg	1,626–1,951 kcal
20 lbs/9.0 kg	575–690 kcal	85 lbs/38.6 kg	1,701–2,042 kcal
25 lbs/11.3 kg	680–816 kcal	90 lbs/40.8 kg	1,776–2,132 kcal
30 lbs/13.6 kg	779–935 kcal	95 lbs/43.1 kg	1,850–2,220 kcal
35 lbs/15.8 kg	875–1,050 kcal	100 lbs/45.3 kg	1,922–2,307 kcal
40 lbs/18.1 kg	965–1,158 kcal	110 lbs/49.8 kg	2,065–2,478 kcal
45 lbs/20.4 kg	1,056–1,267 kcal	120 lbs/54.4 kg	2,204–2,645 kcal
50 lbs/22.6 kg	1,143–1,372 kcal	130 lbs/58.9 kg	2,340–2,809 kcal
55 lbs/24.9 kg	1,228–1,473 kcal	140 lbs/63.4 kg	2,474–2,969 kcal
60 lbs/27.2 kg	1,310–1,573 kcal	150 lbs/68.0 kg	2,606–3,127 kcal
65 lbs/29.5 kg	1,392–1,670 kcal		

Data sourced from: Waltham Center for Pet Nutrition, Burger 1994 and The National Research Council (NRC) 1974

Dogs with Special Needs

A DOG THAT IS COPING WITH DISEASE CAN HAVE VERY specific nutritional requirements related to his/her illness. As a result, special care is essential when formulating a diet

Specialized Nutrition Plans

Specialized nutrition plans can be developed to complement veterinary therapy in treating some medical conditions. These include:

- Low-fat diets for weight reduction and the treatment of pancreatitis

- High-fiber diets for constipation

- Lower-fat diets with suitable levels of fiber for gastrointestinal disorders

- Seniors' diets to reduce the risk of age-related problems in older dogs

- Low-sodium diets to assist in managing congestive heart failure

- Nutrient-dense diets to be fed during recovery from surgery or in the treatment of certain acute or chronic debilitating conditions

intended to address a medical condition. If you are planning to use a home-prepared diet to complement treatment for any disease, it is imperative that you have a full understanding of your dog's nutritional requirements and that you work closely with your veterinarian to monitor the diet's efficacy and safety.

To ensure that a diet is safe, you must consider many factors. The levels of nutrients must be correct — there are some diseases in which specific nutrients can have such significant impact on the health of the dog that there is little margin for error. One example is pancreatitis: a diet for a dog with pancreatitis must be precise in its fat content. If fat levels are too high, the pancreas will continue to overwork, and proper healing will not take place.

Other factors that can influence a diet's safety or efficacy are the ingredients used. As we humans are finding with our own health, some foods can interact with certain medications. A full understanding of foods and their interactions with prescription drugs is imperative if your dog is on a drug regimen for disease treatment.

Due to the gravity of this topic and because such in-depth information on specific illnesses is required, we have not addressed special-needs diets in this book. However, commercial diets formulated to meet the needs of dogs with specific diseases are available through veterinarians. Although a commercially prepared therapeutic diet may not offer optimal nutrition, it should offer safe nutrition. Look for brands that offer high-quality ingredients and work closely with your veterinarian to determine which diet is appropriate for your dog. Your veterinarian will closely monitor your dog's progress on the diet through physical examinations and blood tests. No diet should ever be undertaken for a sick dog without the supervision of a veterinarian.

> ### ✚ DOC'S DOCTRINE
>
> Shedding can be a continuous process for some dogs. Day length and temperature cues stimulate a dog to shed in the spring and fall. Dogs that are kept indoors can miss these cues and may shed continuously.

> ### ✚ DOC'S DOCTRINE
>
> Does your dog routinely vomit after eating grass? You need to see your veterinarian for diagnosis and treatment. The vomiting is a signpost of internal disease.

Puppies and Diet

A HEALTHY DIET IS ESPECIALLY IMPORTANT FOR PUPPIES. Because they are growing, puppies have specific nutritional requirements that must be met in order to ensure that their

When Is Your Puppy Mature?

Although a puppy's most intense period of growth occurs in the first six months of life, the age of maturity varies with breed and/or body type. Usually, the smaller the breed the earlier s/he matures. In general terms, puppies are considered mature at the following times:

- Six to 12 months of age (small to medium breeds)
- Ten to 16 months of age (large breeds)
- Up to 24 months of age (giant breeds)

growth rates are appropriate for their breed and growth curve and that their development is sound. The quality of nutrition received during a puppy's formative period directly influences his/her state of health as an adult.

Compared with adult dogs, puppies must eat a larger quantity of food relative to their size, as they require higher levels of nutrients. This is complicated by the fact that puppies have smaller stomachs, mouths and teeth than full-grown dogs. As a result, puppies must eat smaller meals more frequently: four times a day until they are four months old, then three times a day until they are six months old. At that point, they can be fed twice a day, like adult dogs.

Puppy Nutritional Requirements

A puppy's diet should be nutrient-dense, nutritionally balanced and highly digestible. It's important for young dogs to eat right so their bodies can grow to be structurally sound, with strong bones and muscles. The NRC and the AAFCO have both set guidelines for the minimum levels of nutrients that puppies require for appropriate growth.

Energy Requirements for Puppies Compared with Adult Dogs

Puppies require more energy proportionally than adult dogs until they reach 80% of their adult weight. In general terms, puppies' energy requirements compared with adult dogs are:

- Up to 40% of their adult weight — approximately twice as many calories proportionally
- From 40 to 60% of their adult weight —1.6 times as many calories proportionally
- From 60 to 80% of their adult weight —1.2 times as many calories proportionally

Puppies and Home-Prepared Diets

Since a puppy's diet provides much of the foundation for future health, feeding him/her a home-prepared diet should only be undertaken with the utmost care, understanding and dedication. We have not included puppy recipes, as we feel that the formulation of a home-prepared diet for puppies is a subject worthy of its own book. The mealtime recipes in this book are designed for adult dogs and are not intended for puppies. However, they may be rewarded with home-baked cookies prepared from our recipes.

The safest way to ensure that your puppy receives appropriate nutrition is to feed him/her high-quality food that is specifically designed for puppies — purchase it through your veterinarian or at specialty pet-supply stores.

Choosing the Best Food

Look for the following when choosing a commercially prepared puppy food, and if the information is incomplete on the package, phone the manufacturer with any questions.

- Has met AAFCO minimum standards for growth (or similar criteria)
- Tested through humane feeding trials
- Animal-based protein source, such as chicken, beef or lamb, is the predominant ingredient
- Reputable manufacturer that stands behind its product (look for contact information on the package, including a telephone number)
- Detailed feeding instructions to ensure proper growth rate
- Size-specific formulations (e.g., for small, medium or large breeds)
- Natural preservatives or no preservatives
- Expiry or processed-on date to ensure freshness

A Plump Puppy May Not Be a Healthy Puppy

It is very important not to overfeed your puppy— not only because s/he will be overweight but also because s/he will grow too quickly. Overfeeding predisposes a puppy to growth-related diseases of the bones and joints. Developmental diseases such as hip dysplasia have a direct link to excessive body weight and high growth rate. Another factor in skeletal disease is the over-supplementation of calcium during the developmental stage, which can contribute to skeletal diseases, such as hip dysplasia. But calcium deficiency is another matter (see Just Enough of a Good Thing, below). The damage caused by overfeeding and oversupplementation is usually irreversible and can have serious long-term effects.

Just Enough of a Good Thing

Your puppy requires a fine balance of nutrients to maintain health and promote a safe growth rate. A myriad of health problems result when puppies don't get enough to eat or are fed a diet that is deficient in essential nutrients. For example, chronic protein deficiency causes impaired growth, muscular deterioration, emaciation and, finally, death. A chronic calcium deficiency results in loss of bone density, which is linked to lameness, spontaneous fractures and deviations of the limbs.

Watch and Adjust

Your puppy's diet should be monitored on a weekly basis and adjusted, if necessary, to ensure that s/he is receiving appropriate amounts of energy and nutrients. Your puppy should maintain a lean body composition (a slight layer of fat covering the ribs), have a good coat and maintain a healthy activity level. By four months of age, your puppy should have seen his/her veterinarian three times for vaccinations. Have your veterinarian assess your puppy's body condition at these appointments and make recommendations on feeding patterns.

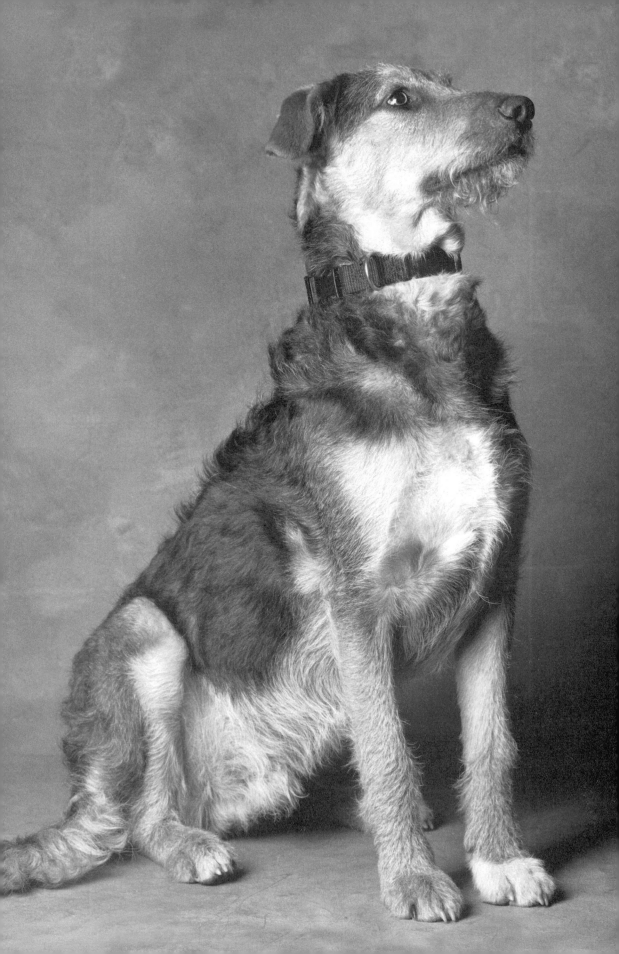

Making It Work

Supporting Wellness

WHILE A NUTRITIOUS DIET IS A KEY COMPONENT OF GOOD health, your dog requires additional support in order to achieve an optimum level of wellness. This support involves not only your own knowledge and powers of observation but also an awareness of situations that may affect your dog's well-being, such as allergies or an inability to tolerate new foods. Working closely with your veterinarian to establish an overall wellness program will also help your dog stay healthy and well. In addition, a wellness program serves as a tool for monitoring how well your dog's diet is working.

> **✚ DOC'S DOCTRINE**
>
> Spear grass (plant awn) is a small dry seedlike object that can burrow into the skin, ears or nose and cause infections or pain. Always check for spear grass after walking or hiking with your dog.

Dogs and New Foods

SINCE MOST DOGS, ESPECIALLY THOSE FED KIBBLE exclusively, have not been exposed to many foods, their digestive systems need time to adjust to new diets. The same common-sense approach parents take to introducing foods to children should be used when feeding new foods to dogs. Introducing new foods gradually, one at a time, helps prevent stomach upsets that new substances might cause. Adding new foods one at a time can also help you identify problem foods. If your dog has an adverse reaction to a food, the most common symptoms are diarrhea, gas and vomiting. These usually occur within 24 hours of ingestion.

> **✚ DOC'S DOCTRINE**
>
> Some dogs pull insistently on their collars when they're on walks. This can damage the dog's throat and make it hard for the person to safely control the dog. A halter device (used for control when walking) is a safe and humane solution to this problem.

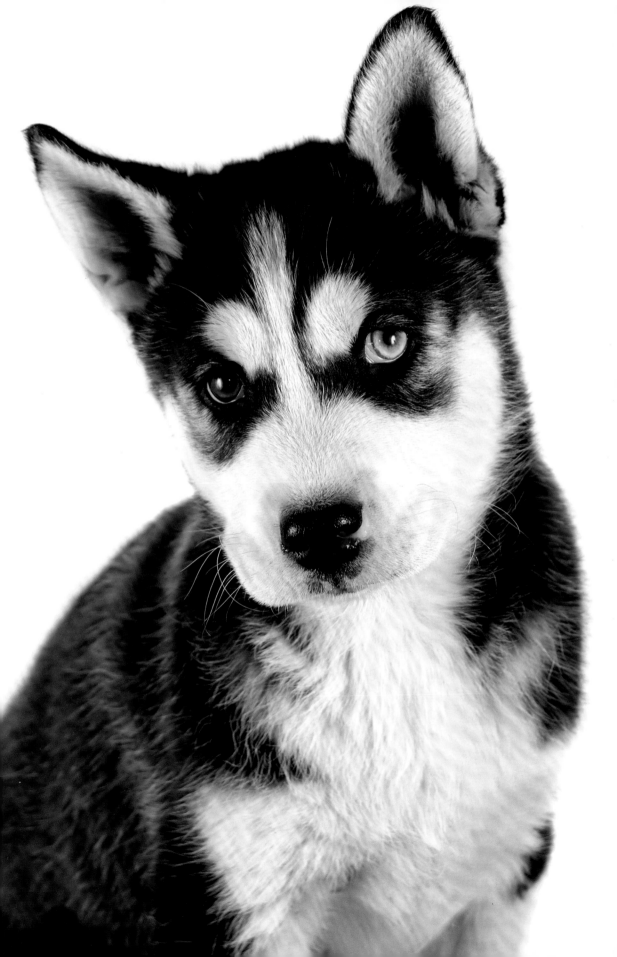

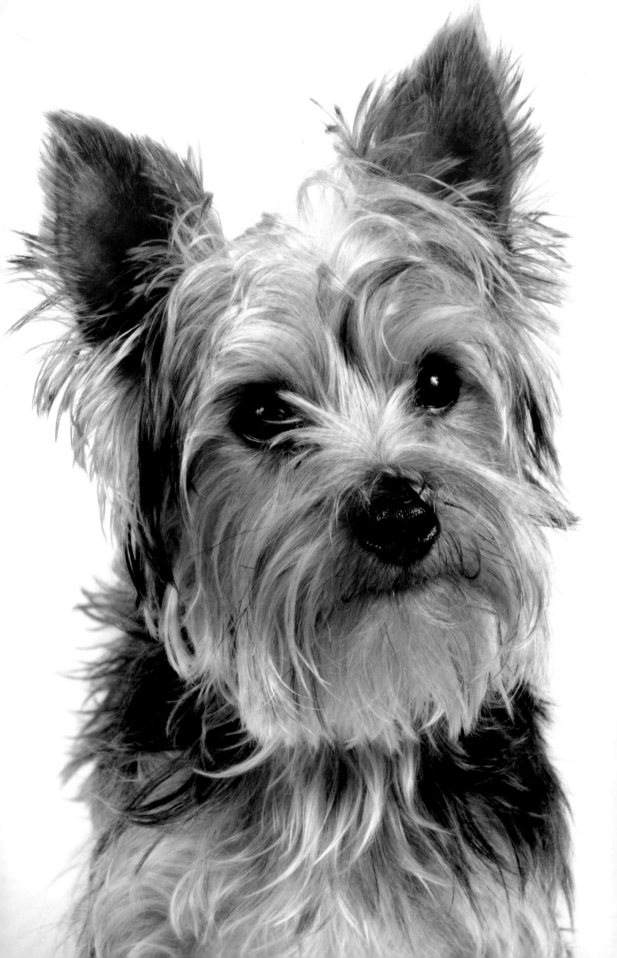

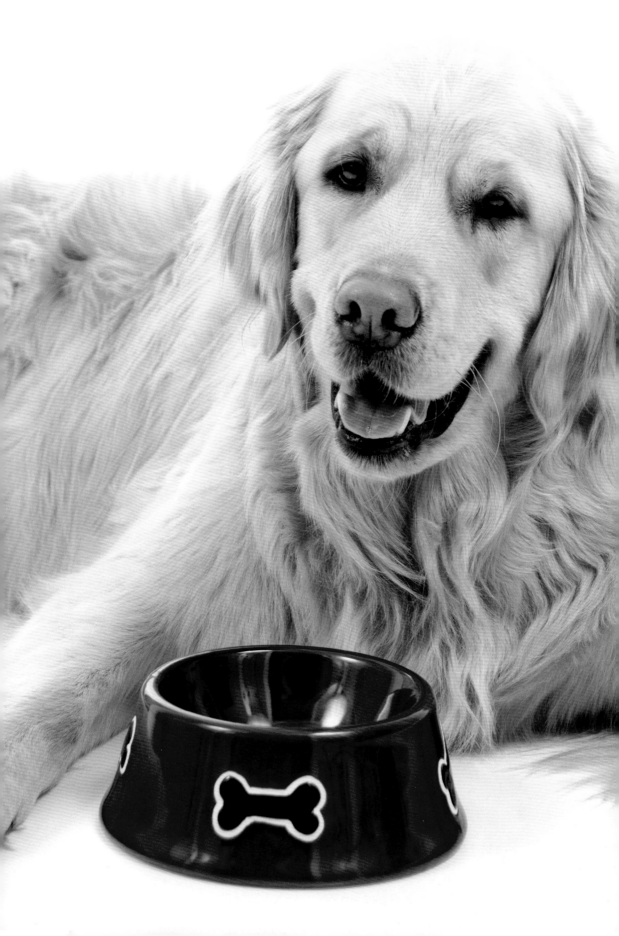

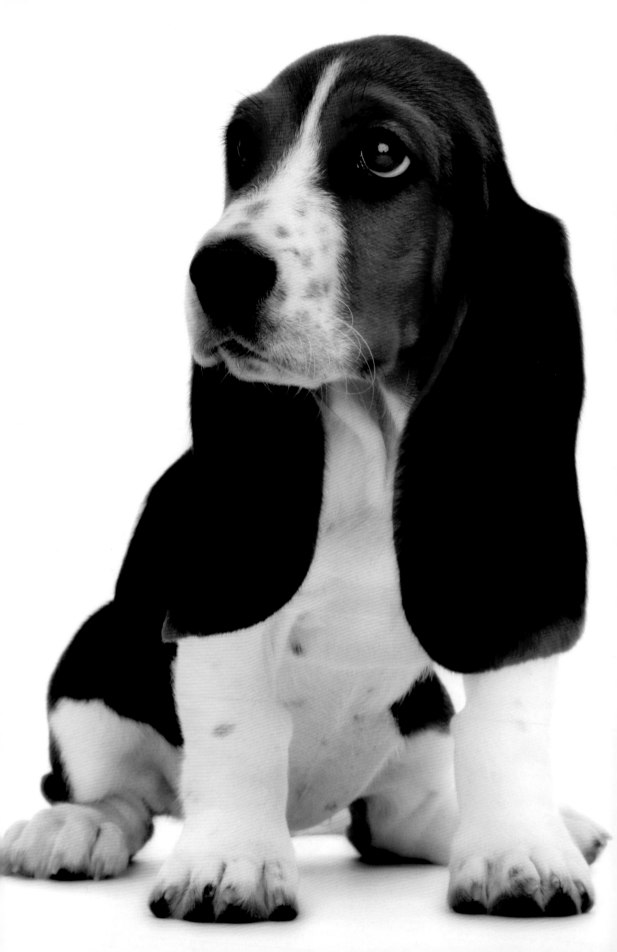

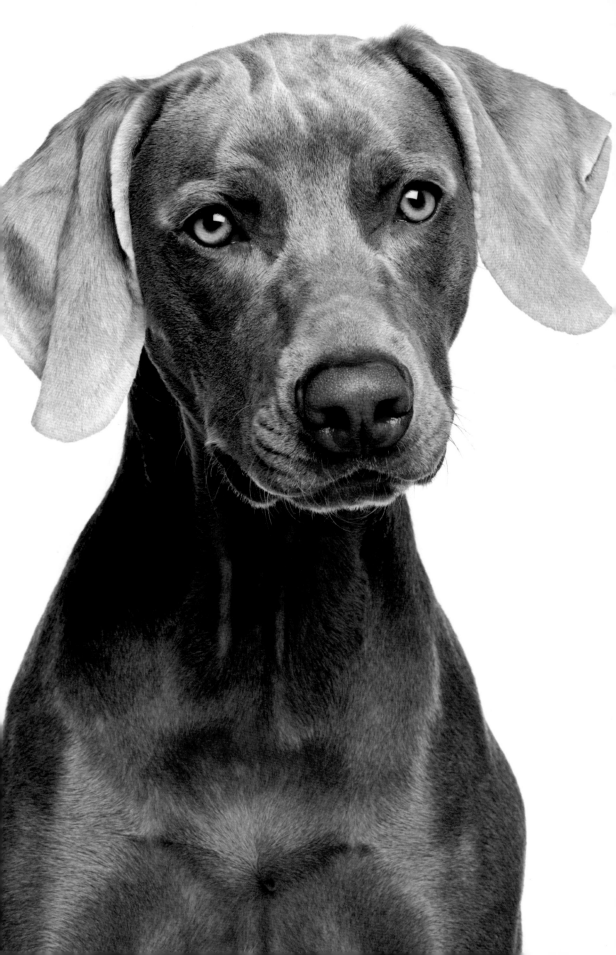

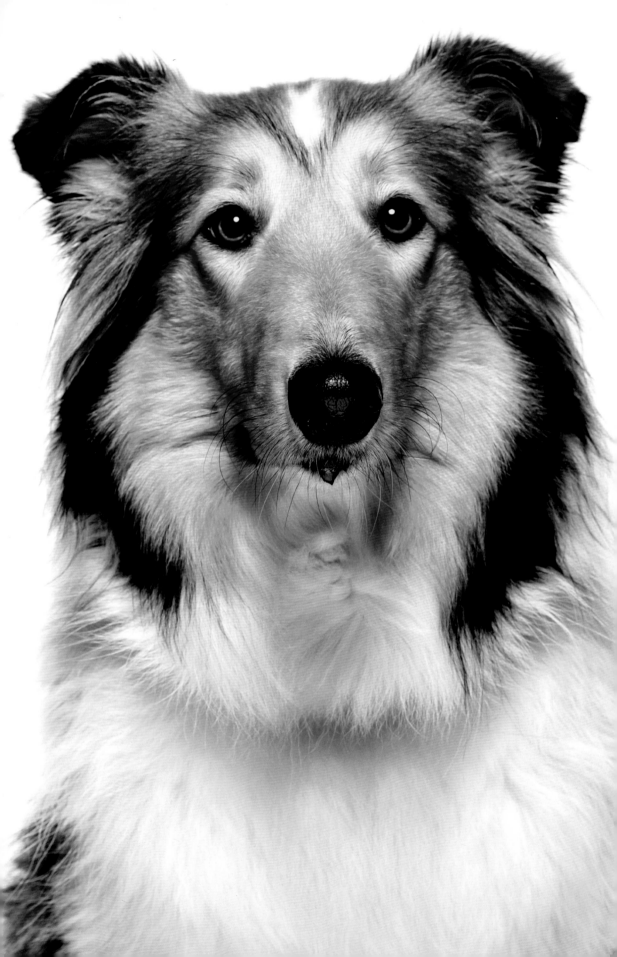

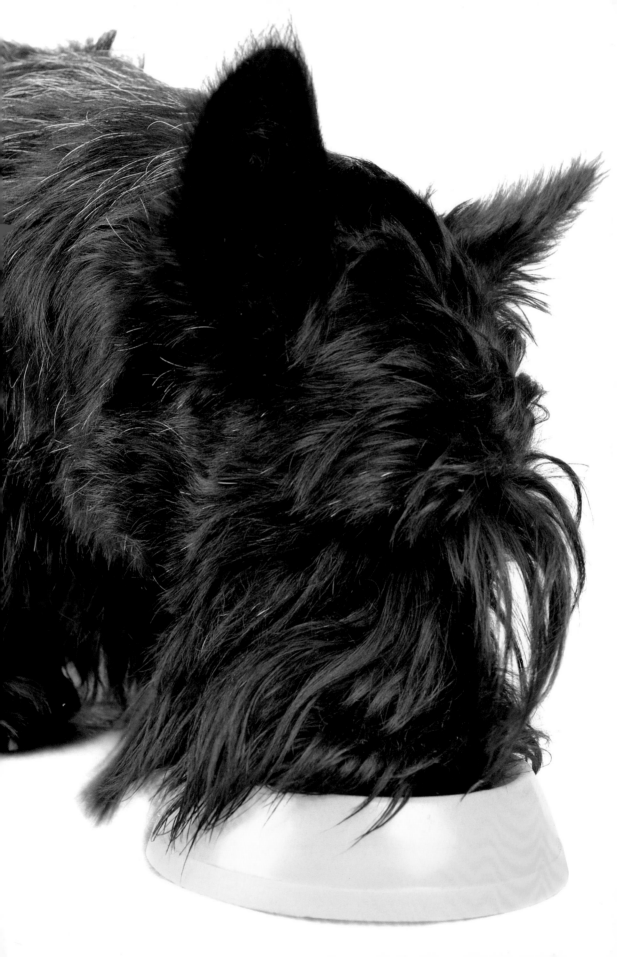

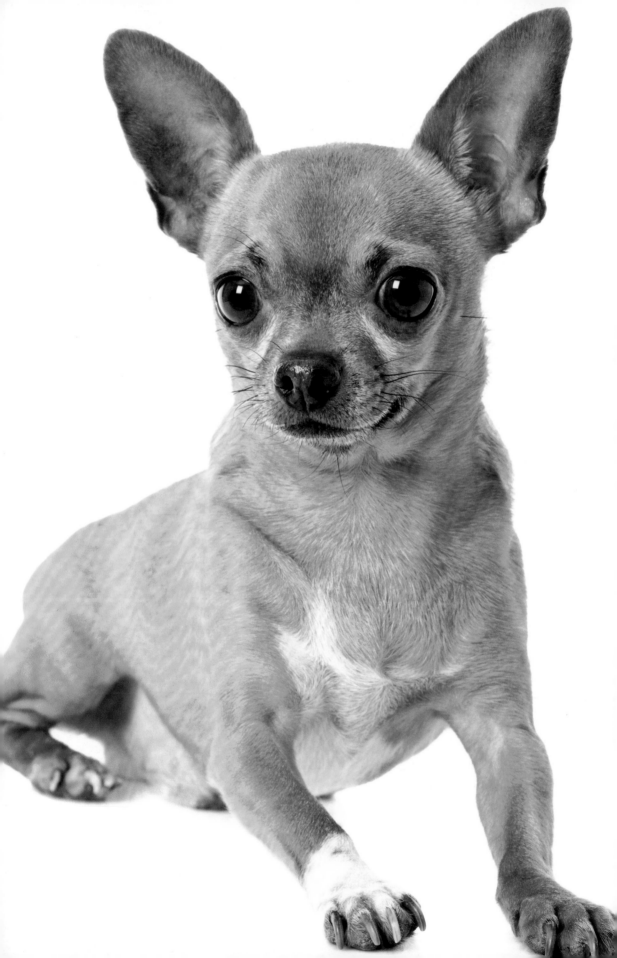

Introducing a Home-Prepared Diet

With the switch from kibble to a home-prepared diet, there is a dramatic change in the texture and digestibility of the food. The gut takes a few days to adapt to these changes, and your dog may have a temporary bout of diarrhea.

To ensure a smooth transition to a home-prepared diet, introduce new foods over an eight-day period. For the first two days, mix 25% of the new food into 75% of the current food. Add cooked brown rice and meat only (no fats, supplements or salts) in the quantities appropriate for your dog (see the Basic Recipe for his/her weight class in Chapter 5). After two days, increase the percentage of new food to 50% and include a vegetable. After two more days, increase the new food to 75% of the total, including the other vegetables or fruits in the vegetable-and-fruit mix. After two days of this combination, increase the new food to 100% and introduce the oil, salts, bonemeal and multivitamin-and-mineral supplement. You can now try using new ingredients, such as other vegetables, meats or grains.

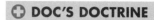

DOC'S DOCTRINE

After hiking with your dog, particularly in the spring and fall, it is very important to check for ticks. Ticks can secrete a neurotoxin that causes hind-limb paralysis. Removal of the tick resolves this problem. To remove a tick, spread the hair away from it, then gently grasp the tick right at the surface of the dog's skin and gently but firmly pull to remove as much of the tick as possible. Wear gloves during removal and wash the tick site thoroughly with soap and water.

Assessing the Diet

You will need to monitor how your dog does on the new diet. No one diet, commercial or home-prepared, is perfect for every dog. Visit your veterinarian and let him/her know you are making significant adjustments to your dog's diet. Watch your dog for any physical or emotional changes and keep track of his/her weight.

Weighing Results

Once you begin feeding a new diet to your dog, you will need to monitor his/her weight regularly to make sure energy needs are being met. Keep an eye on your dog's weight by using a scale or by checking for changes in the amount of fat and muscle over the ribs (see Checking Weight, below).

So long as your dog is in good health, if s/he is losing weight, the reason is simple: there are not enough calories in the diet. That means you'll need to increase the quantity of food your dog receives. Step up the daily caloric intake to that of the next weight class and maintain that regimen for at least two weeks. If your dog stops losing weight after the two-week period, stay at that level. If s/he is still losing weight, move up to the next weight class. Continue to adjust the diet every two weeks until your dog's weight stabilizes.

On the other hand, if your dog is gaining weight, then s/he is eating too much, and you will need to reduce the daily caloric intake. Drop to the weight class immediately below and feed that quantity of food for approximately four weeks. If the weight holds steady, continue to feed your dog that quantity of food.

Why Body Weight Is Important

Both underfeeding and overfeeding will undermine your dog's health. A dog that is too heavy will not be able to tolerate heat and is at increased risk for degenerative joint disease; diabetes; and respiratory, dermatological and orthopedic problems. A dog that is underweight will likely have less energy and a dull, brittle coat. If s/he has lost muscle mass, there may be extra wear on the joints.

Checking Weight

Although you should have your dog weighed regularly at the vet's, between visits you can check his/her weight yourself. If your dog is small enough that you can pick him/her up, one way to determine his/her weight is to first weigh yourself, then step on the scale while holding your dog off the ground. Your dog's weight is the difference between your weight and what the scale says both of you weigh together.

If you don't have a scale, here's an easy way to check your dog's weight: run your fingertips sideways along the dog's rib cage, pressing lightly. There should be a thin layer of tissue covering the ribs, but you should be able to feel them easily. You should not be able to feel any indentations between the ribs. If your dog is underweight, you will be able to feel the individual ribs and indentations between them, with no layer of fat over them. If s/he is overweight, the ribs will be buried deep beneath a layer of fat.

Next, check the wing of the hip (the tip of the bone at the upper part of the hip). There should be a small layer of tissue overlying the bone, which you should be able to feel easily. If your dog is underweight, the hips will feel sharp and not rounded by the surrounding tissue. On overweight dogs, the hips will be hidden under a layer of fat. If you have problems finding your dog's ribs or the wing of the hip, ask your veterinarian for guidance.

Tracking Wellness

TO HELP YOUR DOG STAY HEALTHY, YOU SHOULD ESTABlish a wellness program with your veterinarian. Wellness testing helps you and your veterinarian build a framework for keeping a constant eye on the status of your dog's health and detecting potential problems at an early stage. A wellness program will include twice-yearly physical examinations and different types of blood and urine testing. The number and types of tests your veterinarian does will depend on your dog's age and current health. These tests also help to show if your dog's diet is appropriate or, in certain cases, if deficiencies exist that need to be corrected.

Complete Blood Count (CBC)

The CBC is a valuable test that can be used to assess your dog's health. Among other diagnostic functions, it provides an absolute total count of the white blood cells and the quantities of each type therein. This helps determine your dog's ability to fight infection. The CBC also counts the red blood cells and assesses their shape and color, which can help identify anemia. Anemia can have many causes, including iron or vitamin B6 and B12 deficiencies, which can be corrected with oral supplements or injections in conjunction with diet.

Chemistry Screen

Among other things, the chemistry screen portion of wellness testing provides an indication of cell health, organ function and mineral levels in the blood. An early diagnosis of abnormal mineral levels might lead to adjustments in your dog's diet that could prevent disease in later life.

Know Your Dog as You Know Yourself

Your own powers of observation are among the most important tools you have for keeping your dog well. Since you know your dog better than anyone else, you are in the best position to notice any changes in his/her appetite, stools, behavior, weight, vitality and general appearance. Pay particular attention to behavioral changes, because they can be an important sign of a medical problem, especially in an older dog. Watch your dog for any physical or emotional changes and keep track of his/her weight.

Urine Test

A urine test assesses kidney function and urinary tract health and can detect the presence of metabolic diseases, such as diabetes. A urine test can also detect crystals or sediment in the urine. If crystals are identified, your dog's diet may be altered to encourage the crystals to dissolve.

Touch and Grooming for Wellness

Petting is emotionally rewarding for both you and your dog. It creates a sense of comfort and encourages bonding. Studies have shown that petting your dog can have positive health benefits for you — for example, it can lower your blood pressure. Luckily, petting is also preventive medicine for your dog. Regularly touching and grooming your dog does more than just keep his/her skin and coat healthy; it also helps you notice external changes, such as hair loss, skin lesions, skin growths, lumps under the skin or fleas, that may be suggestive of more-serious problems. In addition, you should periodically check inside your dog's mouth for any lumps or growths. Make a point of sharing this information — even the smallest changes — with your veterinarian.

> **Tip**
>
> In addition to monitoring your dog's overall health, wellness testing is an indispensable tool for assessing the suitability of his/her diet. When feeding your dog a home-prepared or any other diet, we recommend working with your veterinarian to assess its efficacy on an ongoing basis.

Zoee's Jaw

Not long ago, David and Jennifer had an experience that reconfirmed how important it is to check inside your dog's mouth on a regular basis. They found an alarming red lump in the back of Zoee's jaw, which Grant feared might be cancerous. Grant scheduled surgery for the next day and removed the lump. Fortunately, it was benign, and Zoee was soon back to being her delightful and demanding self. She was very lucky. In Grant's experience, people rarely check inside their dogs' mouths, so they fail to notice lumps until it is too late.

Keep Your Eye on the Doggie Doo

Your dog's stool can reveal information about his/her health, as well as the suitability and digestibility of the food s/he is eating. Consequently, it is very important to pay attention to your dog's stool and to recognize the signs that may indicate potential health problems.

A healthy stool should be light to dark brown or reflect the diet composition in color. It should never be bright red or black; that indicates bleeding in the digestive tract, which requires veterinary attention. A healthy stool should have a firm but not hard texture, and the dog should pass it with minimal effort. Larger-than-normal stool may indicate that your dog's diet is too high in insoluble fiber. If this is the case, the fiber content of the diet should be reduced.

Changes in your dog's stool can also indicate potential health problems. These can include food intolerance and allergies, colon problems and bacterial or viral infection.

Tip

Harris, Zoee, Marley, Buffett and Dylan are all fearless and brave dogs. That is, until they get a "cling-on!" This horrifying experience of having a teeny, tiny piece of stool stuck in their fur sends them into a blind panic, desperately seeking out Mom or Dad to remove the offending passenger. When a dog has something hanging from his/her fur, then, by all means, remove it. But if something is hanging out of the rectum, such as a piece of string or grass, DO NOT pull it out. You can damage the rectum if you do. Carefully cut off what is exposed. If s/he cannot pass the rest of it, see your veterinarian.

Constipation

Constipation is a condition in which a dog strains to defecate and produces very dry, hard stools. Constipation can arise from a variety of causes, ranging from a diet that is too low in fiber to colon problems. If your dog is experiencing chronic constipation, consult your veterinarian to determine the underlying cause. Once s/he determines the cause, medical therapy, along with a high-fiber diet, may be recommended.

Diarrhea

Diarrhea can occur for a number of reasons, only some of which are diet-related. Large-bowel diarrhea (colitis) is by far the most common form. Your dog will have a sudden urge to defecate, and there may be bright red blood or mucus in the stool. If bright red blood is present in diarrhea, immediate veterinary care is needed. Large-bowel diarrhea happens most commonly when a dog eats something inappropriate, such as garbage or rotten

Tip

A dog with diarrhea can benefit from taking lactobacillus capsules, which contain healthy bacteria that can help improve digestive function. Lactobacillus capsules are also good for your dog if s/he has been on antibiotics. Do not supplement your dog's diet with yogurt — it can aggravate the diarrhea.

food. Other causes include intestinal parasites or inflammatory diseases of the colon.

In the case of large-bowel diarrhea that contains a small amount of mucus but no blood, it is advisable to withhold food but not water from your dog for 24 hours. Then feed him/her a bland diet of rice and lean meat for 24 to 48 hours. If the symptoms disappear at this point, reintroduce the regular diet. If they haven't, see your veterinarian.

Small-bowel diarrhea is loose or watery stool in large amounts that originates in the small bowel. Symptoms include watery stools, dark brown digested blood, no sudden urges to defecate, and systemic illness, which can be identified by lethargy, vomiting, loss of appetite and not drinking. If your dog shows any of these symptoms, see your veterinarian immediately.

> **✚ DOC'S DOCTRINE**
>
> Tumors on or below the skin can be either benign (good) or malignant (bad). Soft, movable lumps under the skin of older dogs are usually fatty, benign tumors called lipomas. A veterinarian should check all lumps to verify what types of tumors they are and to recommend a treatment plan.

Your Dog's Teeth

Keeping an eye on your dog's teeth and gums and introducing a program of good oral care also has a role to play in his/her health. No matter what type of diet a dog eats, s/he will produce some plaque, and, subsequently, tartar will build up on the teeth. A well-nourished dog is better equipped to fight the progression of plaque and tartar than a dog on a lower-quality diet. Improved nutrition helps strengthen the immune system, which, in turn, helps reduce the level of oral bacteria present, causing less tartar to accumulate on the teeth.

Dental tartar, which is caused by the accumulation of bacteria, can cause gingivitis, or inflammation of the gums. More seriously, if gingivitis is not controlled, it can cause periodontal disease, which may lead to painful abscesses that require surgery or result in tooth loss. If your dog's teeth and gums are in poor condition, s/he may experience pain when chewing, which decreases his/her ability to chew and eat properly. This could lead to digestive problems and diminished nourishment. Moreover, bacteria may enter the bloodstream and cause damage to the liver and kidneys.

A high-quality diet combined with a consistent program of dental hygiene is the best way to decrease tartar buildup and improve your dog's oral health. Brushing your dog's teeth is especially important if s/he is eating a home-prepared diet — unlike hard kibble, the food will not be abrasive enough to scratch off plaque and tartar.

Brushing Your Dog's Teeth

It isn't difficult to brush a dog's teeth, and, with positive reinforcement, it can become an enjoyable routine. You will need a nondetergent toothpaste, flavored for canine tastes, and a specially designed dog toothbrush. Never use human toothpaste, as dogs must to be able to swallow their toothpaste since they cannot rinse out their mouths. Human toothpaste

Feeding Bones

Many people feed their dogs bones as a supplement to regular toothbrushing. However, we do not think this is an absolutely safe practice. Bones can provide the needed abrasion to help keep teeth clean and free of tartar, but they can also be dangerous. If splintered, bones can get caught in the digestive tract, where they can cause a tear or perforation in the walls. This can lead to a life-threatening infection that will require immediate veterinary attention. Although many dogs never have problems eating bones, others have been seriously injured. As it involves potential dangers, feeding bones to your dog is a personal decision.

If you are comfortable with the idea, take the following precautions:

- Use large beef knucklebones, because they are less likely to splinter
- Submerge the bones in boiling water for about 30 seconds to kill surface bacteria and remove excess fat and marrow
- Don't feed bones on an empty stomach
- Don't leave your dog unsupervised with a bone.

contains detergents, and, if swallowed, will likely make your dog sick.

A reward routine is the best way to introduce your dog to dental hygiene. Initially, for a period of two weeks, invite your dog to come to an area specifically desig- nated for brushing his/her teeth. Ask him/her to sit and stay, then offer a food reward when s/he obeys the command. By the third week, your dog will think posi- tively of the experience. At that point, introduce the idea of brushing.

Do not begin with the toothbrush. Rather, place some toothpaste on your index finger or a specially designed finger toothbrush so your dog will become accustomed to the sensation of something running across the outside of his/her teeth. Use gentle circular motions on the outsides of the teeth and the gum line. When your dog is comfortable with having his/her mouth handled, introduce the toothbrush. Use the same gentle circular motions with the brush and, once again, only brush the outside surfaces of the teeth (the movement of the tongue maintains the inside surfaces). Continue offering a food reward to keep the experi- ence positive for your dog.

> ## Cookies
> As home-prepared diets do not offer much abrasion for the teeth, good-quality crunchy cookies should be added to your dog's diet to help with oral hygiene. While they do not replace regular toothbrushing, low-fat, sugar-free cookies can be a healthy and enjoyable dietary addition. We have provided some Licks and Wags cookie recipes in Chapter 6 that provide the hard, crunchy texture that's helpful in maintaining healthy teeth. In our experience, dogs find them delicious.

> ### ✚ DOC'S DOCTRINE
> Keep your dog's toenails short to prevent lameness and ingrown toenails. Trim the nail with dog nail clippers. If you cut them too short and they start to bleed, a cautery stick or direct pressure will help to stop the bleeding.

Exercise

To be happy and healthy and live a long life, your dog needs more than a good diet. S/he also needs the right amount of exer- cise. Exercise helps regulate weight and strengthen muscles, tendons, bones and the cardiovascular system. It aids the digestion process and can improve all bodily func- tions. Exercise may also be a factor in the prevention and maintenance of certain diseases, including diabetes, musculoskeletal diseases and obesity.

Most healthy dogs have abundant energy, and exercise is imperative to their sense of well-being. Dogs that are not able to release their pent-up energy may develop anxiety-related behavioral problems. A sensible exercise routine can diffuse this excess energy and keep your dog well adjusted and his/her appetite healthy.

However, there are health situations in which exercise should be carefully regulated. Dogs with advanced degenerative joint disease (arthritis), cardiac disease or diabetes need to exercise with care. If your dog suffers from any of these conditions, work with your veterinarian to develop a suitable exercise program for him/her.

Overexercising can have negative health effects on obese dogs: it can overwork or damage the joints and stress the cardiovascular system. Introduce an obese dog to an exercise regimen gradually, in conjunction with a weight-loss diet. Healthy dogs should not be overexercised, either. The weekend-warrior syndrome (letting your dog rest all week, then overdoing exercise on the weekend) is not healthy. You should give your dog moderate, consistent exercise throughout the week.

Potential Emergencies and Food Safety

NO MATTER HOW CAREFULLY YOU PLAN AND INTRODUCE your dog's diet and monitor and support its efficacy through wellness testing and the best possible care, there are some potentially dangerous situations that your dog may encounter. These include toxic foods, choking, food allergies and foods that are unsafe due to bacterial contamination. Knowing what to look out for and how to deal with such a situation, should it arise, can prevent your dog from experiencing discomfort. It might even save his/her life.

Food Intolerance and Allergies

Just like people, dogs can be prone to food intolerance and allergies. Food intolerance is a condition that involves various physiological responses but not an allergic reaction. The most common symptoms of food intolerance are diarrhea, vomiting and problems with gas accumulation, such as flatulence or bloating.

Food allergies occur when the immune system reacts inappropriately to certain food components — usually proteins. The digestibility of the proteins often dictates their potential to cause reactions. Allergic disease caused by food is a common affliction in dogs. Pruritus, or itchy skin, is a common symptom of food allergies. This is usually noticed on the dog's flanks, tail, anal area, paws, face and ears. Other symptoms can include diarrhea that contains mucus and, in severe but rare cases, anaphylactic shock.

> ### ⊕ DOC'S DOCTRINE
>
> Has your dog been urinating small amounts frequently or started having accidents in the house? This may be caused by a urinary tract infection (UTI). A UTI is itchy, uncomfortable and can be painful. See your veterinarian for diagnosis and treatment.

> ### ⊕ DOC'S DOCTRINE
>
> Does your dog smell? Body odor is usually caused by oversecretion and accumulation of oil by the glands in the skin. Upgrading the diet, using shampoos containing sulfur, ASA, and coal tar, and supplementing your dog's diet with omega fatty acid supplements prescribed by your veterinarian, can help to control this problem.

A food allergy is obvious when it shows up shortly after a change in diet, but it can also appear insidiously, after a dog has been consuming the offending food for many years. Usually, an allergic reaction occurs after prior exposure to the food, as the immune system needs to become sensitized to an allergen before it can react. The next time the offending food is consumed, the immune system activates against the allergen, triggering memory cells that can invoke a cascade of events that appear as an allergic reaction. If you are trying to stop the allergic reaction, you should put your dog on a diet consisting of foods to which s/he has not been previously exposed.

Anaphylactic Shock

Anaphylactic shock is an acute allergic reaction that causes the small airways in the lungs to constrict, causing breathing difficulty. Untreated, it will quickly lead to death from suffocation. This is an emergency situation. If your dog is in distress and gasping for breath, immediately rush him/her to the veterinarian. You dog will receive an injection of adrenaline (epinephrine) and a corticosteroid.

Elimination Diets

The definitive test for food allergies in dogs is an elimination diet. Before a food allergy can be diagnosed, environmental allergies need to be ruled out. If the allergy symptoms abate with the elimination diet, a diagnosis of food allergies can be made. An elimination diet should not be undertaken without the supervision of a veterinarian.

In the early stages, an elimination diet consists of a protein source (meat) and a carbohydrate source (cooked grains or cooked potatoes) that the dog has not been previously exposed to. The elimination diet is fed exclusively for eight to 10 weeks. No other food should be fed for the duration of the diet. The allergic symptoms should start to abate within two to three weeks. Once the allergic symptoms have abated, you can begin introducing new foods and appropriate supplements at two-day intervals, watching for recurrence of allergic symptoms.

Salt as a Toxin

As previously noted, salt is a necessary nutrient for a dog. However, salt can be toxic if given in excess. Salt has sometimes been used to induce vomiting when a dog has consumed a poisonous substance. We can not stress too strongly that salt should never be used to induce vomiting in a dog. Large doses of salt can cause cerebral edema (swelling of the brain), which leads to severe neurological damage. Symptoms include lethargy, marked behavior changes and pressing the head against objects.

Foods that Are Known to Be Toxic to Dogs

Although dogs are able to eat many of the same foods as people, there are some exceptions. The following is a list of foods that can be dangerous — even deadly — for dogs to consume. Never feed your dog any of the foods on this list.

Toxic Foods

- Onions or onion powder
- Chocolate
- Coffee and all coffee-related products
- Chocolate-covered espresso beans (especially toxic)
- Tea
- Alcoholic beverages
- Macadamia nuts
- Hops (used in home beer brewing)
- Grapes and raisins (including all associated products, such as juice or wine)
- Tomato foliage (leaves and stems)
- Green parts of potato (green peelings, sprouts and foliage)
- Rhubarb leaves
- Avocados
- Pits and seeds from fruits (plum, apricot, peach, apple and some varieties of cherry)
- Bitter almonds
- Moldy or spoiled foods

Source: The ASPCA National Animal Poison Control Center
Telephone: 1-888-426-4435 Web site: www.aspca.org/apcc

Other Potential Problem Foods

Although you should never feed your dog the foods on the above list, many other foods have the potential to cause a negative reaction. Ingredients commonly used by people, including herbs, spices and even some vegetables, may contain naturally occurring toxins. These foods are usually safe, provided that they are not consumed in excess. Even some essential vitamins and minerals can be toxic if ingested in excess. New information on foods is constantly emerging. To stay up-to-date on current information, check periodically with a respected organization such as the ASPCA National Animal Poison Control Center (call 1-888-426-4435 or visit the Web site at www.aspca.org/apcc).

Poisoning and Other Related Emergencies

If you suspect that your dog has ingested a poisonous substance, call your veterinarian immediately. S/he will decide whether the substance ingested is toxic or caustic. This is a very important distinction, as it will determine the immediate action that you will need to take.

If your dog ingests a caustic substance, such as bleach, which will likely cause burns to the digestive tract, DO NOT induce vomiting. Immediate veterinary care is essential.

If your dog ingests a toxic substance, such as rodent poison or chocolate, check with your veterinarian immediately to determine if you should make the dog vomit. If you attempt to make your dog vomit and s/he does not vomit or does not produce much material, then you should rush him/her to the veterinarian.

If your dog ingests a large amount of chocolate or ingests a poison — such as strychnine, which is found in gopher poison and other substances — there is a strong possibility that seizures will result.

Seizures are characterized by leg paddling, muscle tremors, and/or loss of bowel or bladder control. If your dog has ingested a toxic substance and seizures have developed, it means that the toxins have already reached the dog's nervous system. Rush him/her to the veterinarian immediately.

Several products will induce vomiting and should be kept on hand in case of an emergency. Syrup of ipecac is available at most drugstores or pharmacies. To induce vomiting, give your dog ¼ tsp (1 mL) per each 2 lbs (1 kg) of body weight. Liquid dish soap can also be used to make a dog vomit. A few drops on the back of the tongue should be adequate — never exceed this amount. If your dog does not vomit, rush him/her to the veterinarian.

Food Safety

Dogs can get sick from the same foodborne illnesses that affect people, including salmonella and E. coli. You should always practice the same safe food-handling procedures for your dog's food that you follow for your own.

- Check the food for spoilage and discard any that is spoiled.
- Cook meat thoroughly.
- Store raw meat separately from other foods.
- Thaw foods in the refrigerator or microwave and use them immediately. Do not refreeze.
- Sanitize counters, cutting boards and utensils after they have been in contact with raw meats with a mild bleach solution.
- Wash hands frequently and thoroughly when preparing food.
- Do not leave perishable food out for more than two hours; if the temperature is 40°F (4°C) or warmer, dangerous bacteria can begin to grow.
- Store foods safely: transfer leftovers to the smallest possible containers so they will cool more quickly.
- Use leftovers within two days.
- Reheat leftovers to at least 165°F (74°C).
- Keep your refrigerator temperature at less than 40°F (4°C).
- Keep your freezer temperature at 0°F (–18°C) or colder.
- Always keep your dog's food and water dishes clean; wash them after every meal.

Choking

Choking is not uncommon in dogs. The signs of choking include distress, drooling, coughing or gasping sounds, and pawing at the mouth. Any food or treat, even rice, can cause a dog to choke if s/he swallows too much at one time. Your dog might choke from eating too fast or not chewing enough or because s/he has swallowed too large a chunk of food. If your dog eats rapidly, cutting food into bite-size pieces and serving it on a flat surface rather than in a bowl may help prevent choking by slowing down his/her ingestion. If you have multiple dogs, feed them apart from each other to avoid competition over food, which often causes rapid ingestion.

⊕ DOC'S DOCTRINE

If your dog has been injured or is lame, you can lift him/her by placing a blanket or board under his/her body and lifting gently. See your veterinarian immediately to determine the extent of the injury.

If your dog chokes, immediately open his/her mouth and look for anything that may be lodged in the throat. Try to scoop out the blockage with your fingers. If this fails, try using a modified Heimlich maneuver: reach your arms around the dog's chest just behind the ribs and give a strong, sudden squeeze. If you are unable to dislodge the blockage, take your dog to the veterinarian immediately.

When Your Dog Throws Up

Vomiting is defined as a forceful involuntary expulsion of stomach contents through the mouth. It can be stressful — for you as well as for your dog. Vomiting can have many causes, including adverse reactions to food, eating too rapidly, ingestion of foreign material or food intolerance. Chronic illness or disorders of the internal organs can also cause vomiting. These conditions are usually associated with other symptoms, such as loss of appetite, listlessness, lethargy and poor appearance. If you see any of these symptoms along with more than one episode of vomiting, consult your veterinarian immediately.

Eating Grass

Occasionally, your dog may eat grass, then vomit up food or foreign material. Dogs often eat grass to induce vomiting when they have an upset stomach. When they are feeling well, they also consume grass to supplement their diet. If there is only one episode of vomiting and your dog is bright and alert afterward, then simply monitoring his/her condition is sufficient. If there are multiple episodes of vomiting or your dog vomits abnormal products, such as bright red blood or black, tarry material, immediate veterinary care is needed.

> **➕ DOC'S DOCTRINE**
>
> Do not use human shampoo or dishwashing soap to bathe your dog. Using inappropriate shampoos can lead to dandruff and secondary skin infections. Dog shampoos are recommended.

> **➕ DOC'S DOCTRINE**
>
> Dogs cool themselves by panting, not by sweating like we do. It is important that they always have a cool area and plenty of fresh water to keep them from overheating.

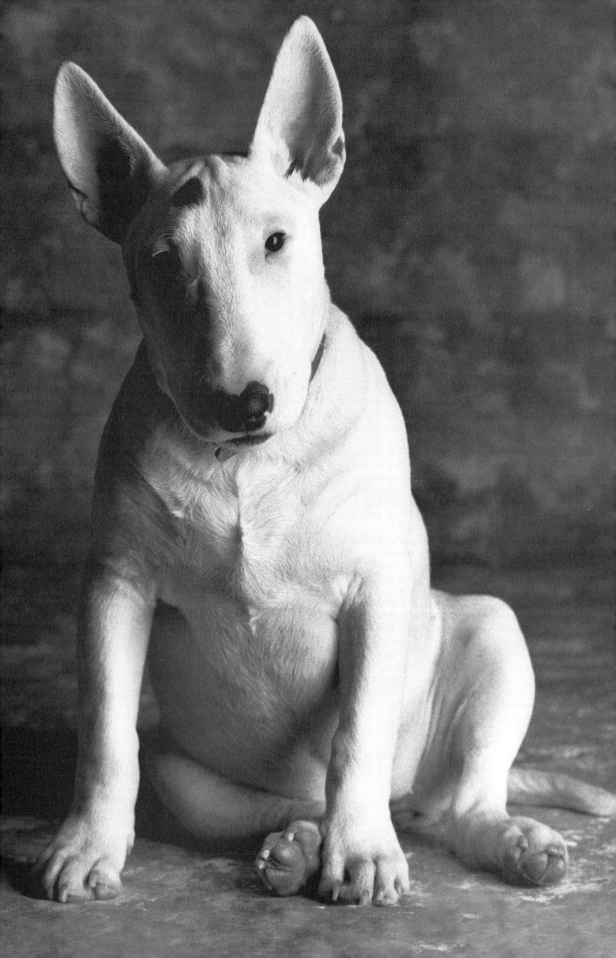

Recipe Basics

Using the Recipes

BEFORE YOU BEGIN MAKING THESE RECIPES FOR YOUR dog, there are a few things you should know. These recipes are intended for use by adult dogs that have no special dietary needs due to state of health or environment (climate) and that are not pregnant, lactating or working dogs. We've taken great care to formulate the recipes and note the required levels of the bonemeal and multivitamin-and-mineral supplements to ensure that the diet provides the full range of nutrients that your dog needs.

The nutritional analysis included with each recipe shows the number of calories and the amounts of protein, carbohydrates and fat it contains. This information comes from *The Nutrient Value of Some Common Foods,* a book published by Health Canada. The nutrient analyses are based on metric measures and weights and on the first ingredients listed where there is a choice. (Variations and optional ingredients are not included.)

All of the recipes are easy to make and have been developed for your convenience, using ingredients that are readily available. Each Basic Recipe contains a vegetable-and-fruit mix. We have provided general instructions for making this mix, along with some sample combinations on page 88. Each Basic Recipe also includes several variations that are based on acceptable protein and carbohydrate substitutions (see charts, page 87). As previously noted, serving your dog a variety of foods over the course of a month helps ensure that s/he receives a good cross section of essential nutrients. Our recommended protein sources are lean ground

Nutrient Analysis

When checking the nutrient analysis of a recipe, you may become concerned about the levels of protein and fat, which often vary among recipes. Please be aware that every recipe provides sufficient levels of these nutrients. Any discrepancy occurs because the recipes have been formulated to meet your dog's daily energy needs (his/her kcal requirement).

If you look at the protein substitutions table on page 87 you'll see that 1 cup (250 mL) of lean ground beef can be substituted with $1^1/_2$ cups (375 mL) cubed chicken breast or $1^2/_3$ cups (400 mL) snapper. All contain approximately 300 kcal. However, since chicken breast and snapper are lower in fat than beef, your dog needs more of these foods to meet his/her energy needs and will, therefore, be getting more protein in a chicken- or fish-based recipe than in one built around beef. Using different meats will cause the protein and fat levels to vary in the recipes, but this variety also helps to ensure that your dog's nutritional needs are met.

beef; lean lamb; chicken or turkey breast; eggs; Atlantic salmon; snapper; and 2% cottage cheese. Our recommended carbohydrate sources are brown rice, pasta and potatoes.

Canola oil and iodized salt are added to most recipes, as is potassium chloride powder. Look for potassium chloride in the salt substitute section of supermarkets or natural-food stores. Human-grade bonemeal and multivitamin-and-mineral supplements are available at specialty pet- or health-food stores (see Chapter 7 to find your dog's needs). If your veterinarian prescribes other therapeutic supplements, give them as directed.

Start with Your Dog's Weight Class

AS EACH DOG IS UNIQUE, INTRODUCE A HOME-PREPARED diet using the recipes for your dog's current weight class (see Introducing a Home-Prepared Diet, page 65, for information on gradually introducing new foods). Then monitor how your dog is doing (see Weighing Results, page 66 and Tracking Wellness, page 67).

Why Weight Matters

Your dog's energy requirements are based on body weight, but it is important to understand that energy needs do not increase in a linear fashion as simple multiples of weight. On a per-pound or per-kilogram basis, the smaller the dog, the more energy s/he needs. For instance, an average dog that weighs 5 lbs (2.3 kg) needs 203 to 244 kcal per day. Based on that information, it might be reasonable to assume that an average dog that weighs 10 lbs (4.5 kg) needs twice as many calories — 406 to 488 kcal per day. In fact, s/he actually needs fewer than that — 341 to 411 kcal per day. Feeding your 10-lb (4.5 kg) dog a double portion of a recipe that is right for a 5-lb (2.3 kg) dog would likely cause him/her to gain weight. And if you randomly reduce the quantity of food by ladling off a spoonful or two, you are throwing off a carefully formulated balance and putting your dog at risk for nutritional deficiencies.

Essentially, larger dogs develop a kind of economy of scale with their energy needs. If they weigh five times as much, they don't need five times as many calories. When using these recipes, stick with the recipes in your dog's weight class, but if s/he loses or gains weight, adjust by moving up or down to the adjacent weight classes.

> **Tip**
> If your dog consumes a milk product without previous exposure to dairy foods, low-level diarrhea may result. To improve his/her ability to tolerate dairy products, add a small amount of yogurt or cottage cheese to any of the Basic Recipes. After a few weeks, your dog should be able to enjoy cottage cheese as a protein substitution.

Follow the Instructions

Each Basic Recipe makes four servings, enough for two days of meals. After you have made the recipe, divide it into four equal servings and feed your dog a one-serving meal, adding the required supplements to the individual portion. Place the remaining three portions in individual containers, cover tightly and refrigerate until you're ready to serve them. If you can't use the remaining servings within two days — for example, if you prepare a gourmet meal for your dog and want to serve that instead of the remaining portions from a Basic Recipe — you can freeze the containers. Defrost them in the refrigerator or microwave and warm them up before serving. Add the bonemeal and multivitamin-and-mineral supplements just before serving.

Vary the Ingredients

As noted, varying the ingredients in your dog's diet not only makes eating more pleasurable, it also helps to ensure that s/he receives a good cross section of essential nutrients. The following tables give the equivalent amounts of our recommended protein and carbohydrate sources to help you add variety to your dog's diet.

Substituting Ingredients

Note: cubes are $\frac{1}{2}$-inch (1 cm).

Protein Substitutions
1 CUP (250 ML) DRAINED COOKED LEAN GROUND BEEF =
•4 large eggs, hard-boiled and peeled
•1$\frac{1}{2}$ cups (375 mL) cubed cooked boneless skinless chicken breast
•1$\frac{1}{2}$ cups (375 mL) cubed cooked boneless skinless turkey breast
•1 cup (250 mL) cubed cooked lean boneless lamb
•1$\frac{1}{4}$ cups (300 mL) cubed cooked boneless skinless Atlantic salmon (on occasion)
•1$\frac{2}{3}$ cups (400 mL) cubed cooked boneless skinless snapper (on occasion)
•1$\frac{1}{3}$ cups (325 mL) 2% cottage cheese
Carbohydrate Substitutions
1 CUP (250 ML) COOKED LONG-GRAIN BROWN RICE =
•1$\frac{1}{8}$ cups (275 mL) drained cooked macaroni
•2$\frac{1}{4}$ cups (550 mL) cubed peeled boiled potatoes

Essential Information

- If using cottage cheese as a substitution, omit salt from the recipe.
- If using turkey or lamb in combination with potatoes, increase the canola oil in the recipe as follows:
  - 5 to 50-lb (2.3 to 22.6 kg) dog, increase by 25%
  - 50 to 150-lb (22.6 to 68.0 kg) dog, increase by 50%
- If using turkey or lamb in combination with macaroni, increase the canola oil in the recipe as follows:
  - 5 to 50-lb (2.3 to 22.6 kg) dog, amounts are OK
  - 50 to 150-lb (22.6 to 68.0 kg) dog, increase by 25%
- If using snapper or cottage cheese in combination with macaroni or potatoes, increase the canola oil in the recipe by 50%.

Vegetable-and-Fruit Mix

When preparing the vegetable-and-fruit mix for the Basic Recipes, use any combination of vegetables, fruits and berries that your dog enjoys and can tolerate and that are safe (see Foods that Are Known to Be Toxic to Dogs, page 76).

In order to ensure that there's enough variety in your dog's diet, we recommend using at least three vegetables and fruits in the mix. If you are using frozen or canned vegetables, choose packages that do not contain added salt.

> **Tip**
> For large dogs or multiple-dog families, you can make larger amounts of these mixes. Cover and store in the refrigerator for up to three days or freeze for up to three months. For smaller dogs, you can divide these recipes.

> **Tip**
> Try combining different vegetables and fruits, especially those that are in season. Remember, vegetables and fruits must be either pureed or cooked so your dog can digest them properly. A good rule is that if the food needs to be cooked for human consumption — corn, for example — it should be cooked for your dog.

Basic Vegetable-and-Fruit Mixes

MAKES ABOUT 1 CUP (250 ML)		
#1		
¼ cup	finely chopped peeled carrot	50 mL
¼ cup	finely chopped ripe tomato	50 mL
½ cup	chopped green beans, cooked and drained	125 mL
Quarter	apple, cored	Quarter
#2		
½ cup	chopped green beans, cooked and drained	125 mL
¼ cup	green peas, cooked and drained	50 mL
¼ cup	corn kernels, cooked and drained	50 mL
¼ cup	blueberries or chopped peeled banana	50 mL

1. In a food processor or blender, combine all ingredients. Puree for about 30 seconds. Use immediately or cover and refrigerate or freeze. If frozen, thaw before using.

Cooking Meats and Fish

Ground Beef
Skillet method: In a nonstick skillet over medium-high heat, cook beef, stirring and breaking up with a spoon, until no longer pink. Drain off fat. Let cool until just warm to the touch.

Microwave method: In a microwave-safe dish, combine 1 lb (500 g) ground beef with 2 cups (500 mL) water. Cover tightly and microwave on High for 3 minutes or until no longer pink. Let cool, covered, until just warm to the touch. Drain off liquid before using.

Chicken and Turkey
Skillet method: Cut boneless skinless chicken or turkey breast into ½-inch (1 cm) cubes. In a nonstick skillet over medium heat, cook cubes, stirring, until no longer pink inside. Let cool until just warm to the touch.

Microwave method: In a microwave-safe dish, combine 1 whole chicken breast (bone in, skin on), split in half, with ¼ cup (50 mL) water. Cover tightly and microwave on High for 7 minutes or until no longer pink inside. Let cool, covered, until just warm to the touch. Remove and discard skin and bones. Drain off liquid. Cut into ½-inch (1 cm) cubes.

Poaching method: Cut boneless skinless chicken or turkey breast into ½-inch (1 cm) cubes. In a shallow pan of simmering water, cook cubes for 5 to 10 minutes (or cook bone-in skin-on chicken breasts split in half in single layer for 15 to 20 minutes) or until no longer pink inside. Drain off liquid. Let cool until just warm to the touch. Remove and discard skin and bones and cut into ½-inch (1 cm) cubes, if necessary.

Lamb
Skillet method: Cut lean boneless lamb into ½-inch (1 cm) cubes. In a nonstick skillet over medium-high heat, cook lamb, stirring, until no longer pink inside. Drain off fat. Let cool until just warm to the touch.

Microwave method: In a microwave-safe dish, combine 2 lbs (1 kg) lean boneless lamb with 1 cup (250 mL) water. Cover tightly and microwave on High for 20 minutes or until lamb is no longer pink inside. Let cool, covered, until just warm to the touch. Drain off liquid. Cut into ½-inch (1 cm) cubes.

Poaching method: Cut lean boneless lamb into ½-inch (1 cm) cubes. In a shallow pan of simmering water, cook lamb for 5 to 10 minutes or until no longer pink inside. Drain off liquid. Let cool until just warm to the touch.

Fish

Microwave method: In a microwave-safe dish, place 6- to 8-oz (175 to 250 g), ½-inch (1 cm) thick boneless fish fillet. Cover tightly and microwave on High for 2½ minutes or until fish flakes easily when tested with a fork. Let cool, covered, until just warm to the touch. Remove skin, if necessary. Cut into ½-inch (1 cm) cubes.

Poaching method: In a shallow pan of simmering water, cook boneless skinless fish fillet for about 10 minutes per inch (2.5 cm) of thickness or until fish flakes easily when tested with a fork. Drain off liquid. Let cool until just warm to the touch. Cut into ½-inch (1 cm) cubes.

> **Tip**
> When purchasing potassium chloride (salt substitute) to add to our recipes, check to ensure that it conforms to the strength we have used: 1,050 mg of potassium per ¼ tsp (1 mL). Be aware that potassium chloride purchased from a pharmacy has a stronger concentration of potassium than salt substitutes.

....

Cooking Carbohydrates

Macaroni

In a saucepan, bring water to a rapid boil. Add macaroni and cook, stirring occasionally, for 8 to 10 minutes or until soft. Drain well and rinse under cool water to prevent sticking. Let cool until just warm to the touch.

Brown Rice

Cook according to package directions. Let cool until just warm to the touch.

Note: ⅓ cup (75 mL) raw rice yields 1 cup (250 mL) cooked rice.

Note: Do not add salt if package directions suggest to.

> **Tip**
> Feel free to substitute the same amount of your favorite fresh pasta and cook according to the package instructions.
> **Note:** If using long noodles, such as spaghetti or linguine, chop them into bite-size pieces before serving.

Potatoes

In a saucepan, bring water to a boil. Add whole unpeeled potatoes and boil gently for about 20 minutes or until tender. Let cool until just warm to the touch. Peel potatoes and discard skins. Cut into ½-inch (1 cm) cubes.

Gourmet Recipes and Treats

DOGS ENJOY DIFFERENT FLAVORS JUST AS PEOPLE DO, SO in addition to basic and nutritious everyday food, we've included a selection of gourmet recipes that, with the added supplements, also meet your dog's nutritional requirements. These delicious breakfasts and dinners use ingredients that you are likely to be preparing for yourself. You can easily set some food aside and make a mouthwatering meal for your dog. We speak from experience when we say that your thoughtfulness will be greatly appreciated.

You can also use the gourmet recipes to develop your skills using flavor boosters. Very small amounts of herbs and spices, such as basil, thyme, tarragon, oregano and garlic, can be added to the Basic Recipes to enhance their flavor. The gourmet recipes will give you an idea of the amounts of these flavor boosters that are appropriate for your dog's weight.

And last, but certainly not least, are treats. Because your dog loves treats, they are helpful in strengthening the bond between the two of you. When they're made from wholesome, natural ingredients, they can also be a healthy addition to his/her diet. In Chapter 6, we are happy to share some of our delicious and nutritious Licks and Wags cookie recipes with you. Our cookies do not contain any sugar, meat products or salt and they have a crunchy texture, which helps maintain good oral health.

A Pinch and a Dash

A number of recipes call for a "pinch" or a "dash" of an ingredient. A pinch is a term used for measuring dry ingredients. It describes the amount of a dry ingredient that can be held between the thumb and forefinger. It equals approximately ¹⁄₁₆ tsp (0.25 mL). A dash is the amount of liquid seasoning that is added to a recipe with a quick stroke of the hand – ⅛ tsp (0.5 mL) or less.

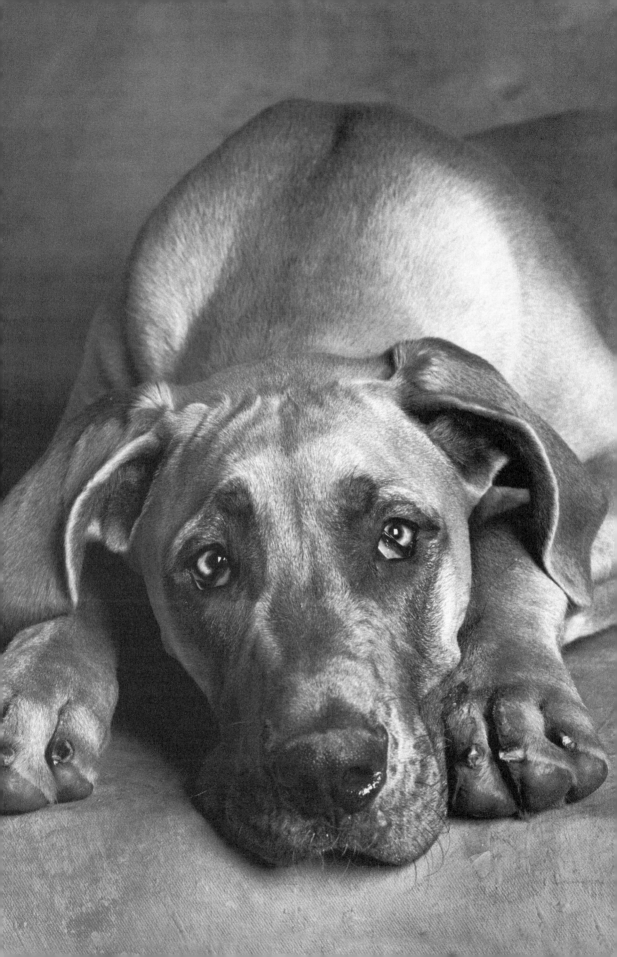

Meals

5 LBS | *2.3* KG

BASIC RECIPE •

Beef and Rice

MAKES 4 SERVINGS

This recipe should be divided into 4 servings, each containing approximately 113 kcal, or half the daily requirement. To meet your dog's nutritional needs, feed 2 servings a day.

¾ cup	cooked long-grain brown rice	175 mL
⅔ cup	drained cooked lean ground beef	150 mL
⅓ cup	pureed vegetable-and-fruit mix	75 mL
1½ tsp	canola oil	7 mL
Pinch	iodized salt	Pinch
Pinch	potassium chloride (salt substitute)	Pinch
	Bonemeal and multivitamin-and-mineral supplements (see Chapter 7, page 198)	

1. In a bowl, combine rice, beef, vegetable-and-fruit mix, oil, salt and potassium chloride. Mix thoroughly. Divide into 4 equal portions.

2. Stir supplements into 1 portion and serve immediately. Cover and refrigerate or freeze the remaining portions. Stir supplements into each portion just before serving.

• •

Tips

For basic instructions on how to cook the meats and carbohydrates, see pages 89 to 91.

For information on how to prepare the vegetable-and-fruit mix, see page 88.

For information on additional protein or carbohydrate substitutions, see page 87.

Cubes are ½ inch (1 cm).

Nutritional Analysis *(Per Serving)*

113 kcal	10.6 g Carbohydrates
6 g Protein	5 g Fat

Variations

- **Chicken and Rice:** Substitute 1 cup (250 mL) cubed cooked boneless skinless chicken breast for the beef.
- **Turkey and Rice:** Substitute 1 cup (250 mL) cubed cooked boneless skinless turkey breast for the beef.
- **Lamb and Rice:** Substitute ⅔ cup (150 mL) cubed cooked lean boneless lamb for the beef.
- **Meat and Macaroni:** Use the appropriate amount of your preferred meat and substitute ¾ cup (175 mL) drained cooked macaroni for the rice.
- **Meat and Potatoes:** Use the appropriate amount of your preferred meat and substitute 1⅓ cups (325 mL) cubed peeled boiled potatoes. Omit potassium chloride.

The daily caloric requirement of a 5-lb (2.3 kg) dog ranges from 203 to 244 kcal.

GOURMET RECIPE •

Cottage Cheese, Fruit and Toast

MAKES 1 SERVING		
Quarter	large hard-boiled egg, peeled	Quarter
Half	slice whole wheat toast, torn into bite-size pieces	Half
2 tbsp	2% cottage cheese	25 mL
1 tbsp	blueberries, thawed if frozen	15 mL
1½ tsp	diced cored apple	7 mL
1½ tsp	chopped peeled banana	7 mL
¼ tsp	canola oil	1 mL
	Bonemeal and multivitamin-and-mineral supplements (see Chapter 7, page 198)	

Tip

If your dog consumes a milk product without previous exposure to dairy foods, low-level diarrhea may result. To properly break down and digest dairy products, your dog needs an enzyme called lactase, which must be developed gradually. To improve his/her ability to tolerate dairy products, add a small amount of yogurt or cottage cheese to any of the Basic Recipes. After a few weeks, your dog should be able to enjoy the calcium-rich foods from the dairy group and will lap up tasty breakfasts, such as Cottage Cheese, Fruit and Toast.

1. In a serving bowl, combine egg, toast, cottage cheese, blueberries, apple, banana, oil and supplements. Mix thoroughly. Serve immediately.

• •

Nutritional Analysis *(Per Serving)*

104 kcal	10.4 g Carbohydrates
7.1 g Protein	3.7 g Fat

GOURMET RECIPE •

Stir-Fried Ginger Beef with Greens

MAKES 1 SERVING

• Wok

½ tsp	canola oil	2 mL
3 tbsp	cubed (½ inch/1 cm) top sirloin steak	45 mL
⅛ tsp	minced gingerroot	0.5 mL
Pinch	minced garlic	Pinch
1 tbsp	chopped green beans, thawed if frozen	15 mL
1½ tsp	green peas, thawed if frozen	7 mL
1½ tsp	finely chopped spinach	7 mL
½ tsp	light soy sauce	2 mL
2½ tbsp	cooked long-grain brown rice	32 mL
	Bonemeal and multivitamin-and-mineral supplements (see Chapter 7, page 198)	

1. In a wok or small nonstick skillet, heat oil over medium heat. Add steak, ginger and garlic. Cook, stirring, until steak is no longer pink inside. Add green beans, peas, spinach and soy sauce. Cook, stirring frequently, for 4 minutes or until vegetables are soft. Transfer to a serving bowl.

2. Add rice. Let cool until just warm to the touch. Stir in supplements. Serve immediately.

• •

Nutritional Analysis *(Per Serving)*

109 kcal	8.8 g Carbohydrates
8.1 g Protein	4.5 g Fat

GOURMET RECIPE •

Salmon and Dill Pasta

MAKES 1 SERVING

½ tsp	canola oil	2 mL
3 tbsp	cubed (½ inch/1 cm) boneless skinless salmon	45 mL
1 tbsp	finely chopped tomato	15 mL
1 tbsp	finely chopped zucchini	15 mL
2 tsp	finely chopped spinach	10 mL
2 tsp	tomato sauce	10 mL
Pinch	dried dillweed	Pinch
Pinch	minced garlic	Pinch
3 tbsp	drained cooked rotini or macaroni	45 mL
	Bonemeal and multivitamin-and-mineral supplements (see Chapter 7, page 198)	

1. In a small saucepan, heat oil over medium-low heat. Add salmon and cook, stirring, until fish flakes easily when tested with a fork. Add tomato, zucchini, spinach, tomato sauce, dill and garlic. Cook, stirring, for 5 minutes or until vegetables are soft. Transfer to a serving bowl. Add rotini and mix thoroughly. Let cool until just warm to the touch.

2. Stir in supplements. Serve immediately.

• •

Nutritional Analysis *(Per Serving)*

120 kcal	9.7 g Carbohydrates
8.9 g Protein	5 g Fat

Buffett's Tale
When David and Jennifer adopted Buffett, he was quite sick and terribly emaciated. They had a difficult time getting him to eat, then they tried salmon, which he loved. He enjoyed it so much that they developed this recipe for him. It quickly became his favorite meal. Buffett is still a little finicky about food, but bring on the fish and he's transported to culinary heaven.

BASIC RECIPE •

Chicken and Rice

MAKES 4 SERVINGS		

This recipe should be divided into 4 servings, each containing approximately 185 kcal, or half the daily requirement. To meet your dog's nutritional needs, feed 2 servings a day.

1½ cups	cubed cooked boneless skinless chicken breast	375 mL
1⅓ cups	cooked long-grain brown rice	325 mL
½ cup	pureed vegetable-and-fruit mix	125 mL
2 tsp	canola oil	10 mL
⅛ tsp	iodized salt	0.5 mL
⅛ tsp	potassium chloride (salt substitute)	0.5 mL
	Bonemeal and multivitamin-and-mineral supplements (see Chapter 7, page 198)	

Tips

For basic instructions on how to cook the meats and carbohydrates, see pages 89 to 91.

For information on how to prepare the vegetable-and-fruit mix, see page 88.

For information on additional protein or carbohydrate substitutions, see page 87.

Cubes are ½ inch (1 cm).

The daily caloric requirement of a 10-lb (4.5 kg) dog ranges from 341 to 411 kcal.

1. In a bowl, combine chicken, rice, vegetable-and-fruit mix, oil, salt and potassium chloride. Mix thoroughly. Divide into 4 equal portions.

2. Stir supplements into 1 portion and serve immediately. Cover and refrigerate or freeze the remaining portions. Stir supplements into each portion just before serving.

• •

Nutritional Analysis *(Per Serving)*

185 kcal	18.6 g Carbohydrates
17 g Protein	4 g Fat

Variations

- **Beef and Rice:** Substitute 1 cup (250 mL) drained cooked lean ground beef for the chicken.
- **Turkey and Rice:** Substitute 1½ cups (375 mL) cubed cooked boneless skinless turkey breast for the chicken.
- **Lamb and Rice:** Substitute 1 cup (250 mL) cubed cooked lean boneless lamb for the chicken.
- **Meat and Macaroni:** Use the appropriate amount of your preferred meat and substitute 1¼ cups (300 mL) drained cooked macaroni for the rice.
- **Meat and Potatoes:** Use the appropriate amount of your preferred meat and substitute 2 cups (500 mL) cubed peeled boiled potatoes for the rice. Omit potassium chloride.

GOURMET RECIPE •

Oatmeal, Yogurt and Fruit

MAKES 1 SERVING

½ cup	cooked rolled oats	125 mL
⅓ cup	non-fat yogurt	75 mL
2 tbsp	2% cottage cheese	25 mL
2 tbsp	blueberries, thawed if frozen	25 mL
1 tbsp	diced cored apple	15 mL
1 tbsp	chopped peeled banana	15 mL
½ tsp	canola oil	2 mL
Pinch	potassium chloride (salt substitute)	Pinch
	Bonemeal and multivitamin-and-mineral supplements (see Chapter 7, page 198)	

Tip

If your dog consumes a milk product without previous exposure to dairy foods, low-level diarrhea may result. To properly break down and digest dairy products, your dog needs an enzyme called lactase, which must be developed gradually. To improve his/her ability to tolerate dairy products, add a small amount of yogurt or cottage cheese to any of the Basic Recipes. After a few weeks, your dog should be able to enjoy the calcium-rich foods from the dairy group and will lap up tasty breakfasts, such as Oatmeal, Yogurt and Fruit.

1. In a serving bowl, combine oats, yogurt, cottage cheese, blueberries, apple, banana, oil, potassium chloride and supplements. Mix thoroughly. Serve immediately.

• •

Nutritional Analysis *(Per Serving)*

183 kcal	**23.7 g Carbohydrates**
12.4 g Protein	**4.8 g Fat**

Breakfast of Champions

Don't be surprised if your dog likes breakfast cereal as much as you do. When Judith, our editor, was growing up, her mother cooked oatmeal for the family in the morning and always made an extra bowl for their dog, Butch, which she served with milk. After lapping it up, Butch would ask to go out, then run down the lane to visit Judith's grandmother, who was just a few doors away. It took a while to learn the reason for these regular morning trips. Turns out Granny always made oatmeal, too. But she served hers with cream — Butch's preferred version. We recommend skim milk.

GOURMET RECIPE •

Beef Stew

MAKES 1 SERVING

½ tsp	canola oil	2 mL
5 tbsp	cubed (½ inch/1 cm) top sirloin steak	70 mL
½ cup	cubed (½ inch/1 cm) peeled potatoes	125 mL
½ cup	water	125 mL
⅛ tsp	minced garlic	0.5 mL
Pinch	dried thyme leaves	Pinch
Pinch	iodized salt	Pinch
2 tbsp	green peas, thawed if frozen	25 mL
1½ tbsp	finely chopped carrot	22 mL
1 tbsp	chopped celery	15 mL
	Bonemeal and multivitamin-and-mineral supplements (see Chapter 7, page 198)	

1. In a small saucepan, heat oil over medium heat. Add steak and cook, stirring, until browned. Add potatoes, water, garlic, thyme and salt. Cover and bring to a boil. Reduce heat, cover and simmer for 10 minutes or until potatoes are almost tender.

2. Stir in peas, carrot and celery. Simmer, uncovered, for 10 minutes or until vegetables are soft. Let cool until just warm to the touch.

3. Stir in supplements. Transfer to a serving bowl. Serve immediately.

• •

Nutritional Analysis *(Per Serving)*

180 kcal	19 g Carbohydrates
13.8 g Protein	5.2 g Fat

GOURMET RECIPE •

Tomato and Chicken Rotini

MAKES 1 SERVING		
½ tsp	canola oil	2 mL
⅓ cup	cubed (½ inch/1 cm) boneless skinless chicken thighs	75 mL
2 tbsp	finely chopped tomato	25 mL
1 tbsp	finely chopped zucchini	15 mL
1 tbsp	tomato sauce	15 mL
1½ tsp	finely chopped green bell pepper	7 mL
⅛ tsp	minced garlic	0.5 mL
Pinch	dried basil leaves	Pinch
Pinch	dried oregano leaves	Pinch
⅓ cup	drained cooked rotini	75 mL
Pinch	potassium chloride (salt substitute)	Pinch
	Bonemeal and multivitamin-and-mineral supplements (see Chapter 7, page 198)	

1. In a small saucepan, heat oil over medium heat. Add chicken and cook, stirring, until no longer pink inside. Stir in tomato, zucchini, tomato sauce, green pepper, garlic, basil and oregano. Cover and cook, stirring occasionally, for 10 minutes or until vegetables are soft.

2. Transfer to a serving bowl. Add rotini and mix thoroughly. Let cool until just warm to the touch. Stir in potassium chloride and supplements. Serve immediately.

• •

Nutritional Analysis *(Per Serving)*

193 kcal	18.8 g Carbohydrates
14.4 g Protein	5.6 g Fat

15 LBS | *6.8* KG

BASIC RECIPE •

Turkey and Rice

MAKES 4 SERVINGS

This recipe should be divided into 4 servings, each containing approximately 234 kcal, or half the daily requirement. To meet your dog's nutritional needs, feed 2 servings a day.

2 cups	cubed cooked boneless skinless turkey breast	500 mL
1½ cups	cooked long-grain brown rice	375 mL
1 cup	pureed vegetable-and-fruit mix	250 mL
1 tbsp	canola oil	15 mL
⅛ tsp	iodized salt	0.5 mL
⅛ tsp	potassium chloride (salt substitute)	0.5 mL
	Bonemeal and multivitamin-and-mineral supplements (see Chapter 7, page 199)	

Tips

For basic instructions on how to cook the meats and carbohydrates, see pages 89 to 91.

For information on how to prepare the vegetable-and-fruit mix, see page 88.

For information on additional protein or carbohydrate substitutions, see page 87.

Cubes are ½ inch (1 cm).

1. In a bowl, combine turkey, rice, vegetable-and-fruit mix, oil, salt and potassium chloride. Mix thoroughly. Divide into 4 equal portions.

2. Stir supplements into 1 portion and serve immediately. Cover and refrigerate or freeze the remaining portions. Stir supplements into each portion just before serving.

• •

Nutritional Analysis *(Per Serving)*

234 kcal	22.3 g Carbohydrates
20.9 g Protein	5.9 g Fat

The daily caloric requirement of a 15-lb (6.8 kg) dog ranges from 463 to 556 kcal.

Variations

- **Beef and Rice:** Substitute 1⅓ cups (325 mL) drained cooked lean ground beef for the turkey.
- **Chicken and Rice:** Substitute 2 cups (500 mL) cubed cooked boneless skinless chicken breast for the turkey.
- **Lamb and Rice:** Substitute 1½ cups (375 mL) cubed cooked lean boneless lamb for the turkey.
- **Meat and Macaroni:** Use the appropriate amount of your preferred meat and substitute 1⅓ cups (325 mL) drained cooked macaroni for the rice.
- **Meat and Potatoes:** Use the appropriate amount of your preferred meat and substitute 2½ cups (625 mL) cubed peeled boiled potatoes for the rice. Omit potassium chloride.

GOURMET RECIPE •

Cottage Cheese, Fruit and Toast

MAKES 1 SERVING			
	1	large hard-boiled egg, peeled and chopped	1
	1	slice whole wheat toast, torn into bite-size pieces	1
	¼ cup	2% cottage cheese	50 mL
	2 tbsp	blueberries, thawed if frozen	25 mL
	1 tbsp	diced cored apple	15 mL
	1 tbsp	chopped peeled banana	15 mL
	½ tsp	canola oil	2 mL
	Pinch	potassium chloride (salt substitute)	Pinch

Bonemeal and multivitamin-and-mineral supplements (see Chapter 7, page 199)

Tip

If your dog consumes a milk product without previous exposure to dairy foods, low-level diarrhea may result. To properly break down and digest dairy products, your dog needs an enzyme called lactase, which must be developed gradually. To improve his/her ability to tolerate dairy products, add a small amount of yogurt or cottage cheese to any of the Basic Recipes. After a few weeks, your dog should be able to enjoy the calcium-rich foods from the dairy group and will lap up tasty breakfasts, such as Cottage Cheese, Fruit and Toast.

1. In a serving bowl, combine egg, toast, cottage cheese, blueberries, apple, banana, oil, potassium chloride and supplements. Mix thoroughly. Serve immediately.

• •

Nutritional Analysis *(Per Serving)*

248 kcal	21.5 g Carbohydrates
17.3 g Protein	11.2 g Fat

GOURMET RECIPE •

Texas-Style Chili

MAKES 1 SERVING

⅓ cup	drained cooked lean ground beef	75 mL
1 tbsp	finely chopped tomato	15 mL
1 tbsp	corn kernels, thawed if frozen	15 mL
1 tbsp	tomato sauce	15 mL
1 tsp	finely chopped green bell pepper	5 mL
½ tsp	chopped cilantro	2 mL
½ tsp	canola oil	2 mL
⅛ tsp	minced garlic	0.5 mL
Pinch	chili powder	Pinch
Dash	fresh lime juice	Dash
⅓ cup	cooked long-grain brown rice	75 mL
Pinch	potassium chloride (salt substitute)	Pinch
	Bonemeal and multivitamin-and-mineral supplements (see Chapter 7, page 199)	

1. In a saucepan, combine ground beef, tomato, corn, tomato sauce, green pepper, cilantro, oil, garlic, chili powder and lime juice. Cook over medium heat, stirring occasionally, for 10 minutes or until vegetables are soft. Remove from heat. Stir in rice. Let cool until just warm to the touch.

2. Stir in potassium chloride and supplements. Transfer to a serving bowl. Serve immediately.

• •

Nutritional Analysis *(Per Serving)*

251 kcal	24.2 g Carbohydrates
14.7 g Protein	10 g Fat

Give the Beans a Pass

Even though we haven't used chunks of beef round, we call this Texas-Style Chili. That's because, like Texans, we've left out the beans — in our case because some legumes are toxic to dogs.

Red Snapper Stew

MAKES 1 SERVING	1 ½ tsp	canola oil	7 mL
	½ cup	cubed (½ inch/1 cm) boneless skinless red snapper	125 mL
	¾ cup	cubed (½ inch/1 cm) peeled potatoes	175 mL
	½ cup	water	125 mL
	2 tbsp	chopped green beans, thawed if frozen	25 mL
	2 tbsp	green peas, thawed if frozen	25 mL
	1 tbsp	finely chopped carrot	15 mL
	⅛ tsp	minced garlic	0.5 mL
	Pinch	iodized salt	Pinch
	Pinch	dried tarragon, thyme or basil leaves	Pinch
		Bonemeal and multivitamin-and-mineral supplements (see Chapter 7, page 199)	

1. In a saucepan, heat oil over medium-low heat. Add snapper and cook, stirring, until lightly browned. Add potatoes, water, green beans, peas, carrot, garlic, salt and tarragon. Increase heat to medium. Cover and cook, stirring occasionally, for 10 minutes or until potatoes are tender. Let cool until just warm to the touch.

2. Stir in supplements. Transfer to a serving bowl. Serve immediately.

• •

Nutritional Analysis *(Per Serving)*

275 kcal	27.1 g Carbohydrates
23 g Protein	8.4 g Fat

IF YOUR DOG WEIGHS

20 LBS | 9.0 KG

BASIC RECIPE •

Lamb and Rice

MAKES 4 SERVINGS

This recipe should be divided into 4 servings, each containing approximately 311 kcal, or half the daily requirement. To meet your dog's nutritional needs, feed 2 servings a day.

Tips

For basic instructions on how to cook the meats and carbohydrates, see pages 89 to 91.

For information on how to prepare the vegetable-and-fruit mix, see page 88.

For information on additional protein or carbohydrate substitutions, see page 87.

Cubes are $1/2$ inch (1 cm).

> The daily caloric requirement of a 20-lb (9.0 kg) dog ranges from 575 to 690 kcal.

2 cups	cooked long-grain brown rice	500 mL
1¾ cups	cubed cooked lean boneless lamb	425 mL
1⅓ cups	pureed vegetable-and-fruit mix	325 mL
1½ tbsp	canola oil	22 mL
¼ tsp	iodized salt	1 mL
¼ tsp	potassium chloride (salt substitute)	1 mL
	Bonemeal and multivitamin-and-mineral supplements (see Chapter 7, page 199)	

1. In a bowl, combine rice, lamb, vegetable-and-fruit mix, oil, salt and potassium chloride. Mix thoroughly. Divide into 4 equal portions.

2. Stir supplements into 1 portion and serve immediately. Cover and refrigerate or freeze the remaining portions. Stir supplements into each portion just before serving.

• •

Nutritional Analysis *(Per Serving)*

311 kcal	**29.9 g Carbohydrates**
21.5 g Protein	**11.5 g Fat**

Variations

• **Beef and Rice:** Substitute 1⅔ cups (400 mL) drained cooked lean ground beef for the lamb.

• **Chicken and Rice:** Substitute 2½ cups (625 mL) cubed cooked boneless skinless chicken breast for the lamb.

• **Turkey and Rice:** Substitute 2½ cups (625 mL) cubed cooked boneless skinless turkey breast for the lamb.

• **Meat and Macaroni:** Use the appropriate amount of your preferred meat and substitute 2¼ cups (550 mL) drained cooked macaroni for the rice.

• **Meat and Potatoes:** Use the appropriate amount of your preferred meat and substitute 3½ cups (825 mL) cubed peeled boiled potatoes for the rice. Omit potassium chloride.

GOURMET RECIPE •

Scrambled Eggs with Whole Wheat Toast

MAKES 1 SERVING			
1 tsp	canola oil		5 mL
¼ cup	finely chopped tomato		50 mL
1½ tsp	finely chopped green bell pepper		7 mL
⅛ tsp	minced garlic		0.5 mL
2	large eggs, beaten		2
1½	slices whole wheat toast, torn into bite-size pieces		1½
Pinch	potassium chloride (salt substitute)		Pinch
	Bonemeal and multivitamin-and-mineral supplements (see Chapter 7, page 199)		

1. In a small nonstick skillet, heat oil over medium heat. Add tomato, green pepper and garlic. Cook, stirring, for 5 minutes or until vegetables are soft. Add eggs and cook, stirring, until eggs are just set. Let cool until just warm to the touch.

2. In a serving bowl, combine egg mixture, toast, potassium chloride and supplements. Mix thoroughly. Serve immediately.

• •

Nutritional Analysis *(Per Serving)*

319 kcal	24.9 g Carbohydrates
17 g Protein	16.5 g Fat

GOURMET RECIPE •

Barbecued Hamburgers

MAKES 1 SERVING

• *Preheat barbecue*

½ cup	lean ground beef	125 mL
1	whole wheat hamburger bun	1
¼ cup	finely chopped tomato	50 mL
¼ cup	finely chopped lettuce	50 mL
1 tsp	canola oil	5 mL
	Bonemeal and multivitamin-and-mineral supplements (see Chapter 7, page 199)	

1. Form beef into one ½-inch (1 cm) thick patty. Place on preheated barbecue and grill, turning once, until no longer pink inside. Let cool until just warm to the touch.

2. Cut burger and bun into bite-size pieces. In a serving bowl, combine burger, bun, tomato, lettuce, oil and supplements. Mix thoroughly. Serve immediately.

• •

Nutritional Analysis *(Per Serving)*

346 kcal	29 g Carbohydrates
22.1 g Protein	15.9 g Fat

Zoee's Score

David and Jennifer's dog Zoee planted the idea of making barbecued hamburgers for four-legged family members. One evening, they invited friends to a barbecue. Just as they were getting ready to eat, a guest set his plate on a table and went into the kitchen. Zoee quickly concluded that opportunity was knocking. She calmly strolled over to the table, lifted up the top half of the bun with her nose and extracted the beef patty. As she walked past the guest with the burger in her mouth, he laughed and commented on how cute she looked. Of course, he hadn't yet realized that she'd made off with his dinner.

GOURMET RECIPE •

Basil Chicken and Vegetable Pasta

MAKES 1 SERVING		
1 tsp	canola oil	5 mL
2/3 cup	cubed (1/2 inch/1 cm) boneless skinless chicken breast	150 mL
1/8 tsp	minced garlic	0.5 mL
3 tbsp	finely chopped tomato	45 mL
3 tbsp	finely chopped zucchini	45 mL
2 tsp	finely chopped green bell pepper	10 mL
2/3 cup	drained cooked rotini or macaroni	150 mL
1 tsp	finely chopped fresh basil leaves (or 1/4 tsp/1 mL dried basil leaves)	5 mL
Pinch	iodized salt	Pinch
1/4 tsp	freshly grated Parmesan cheese (optional)	1 mL
	Bonemeal and multivitamin-and-mineral supplements (see Chapter 7, page 199)	

1. In a nonstick skillet, heat oil over medium heat. Add chicken and garlic. Cook, stirring, until chicken is no longer pink. Add tomato, zucchini and green pepper. Cook, stirring, for 6 minutes or until vegetables are soft.

2. Remove from heat and stir in rotini, basil and salt. Sprinkle with Parmesan cheese, if using. Let cool until just warm to the touch.

3. Stir in supplements. Transfer to a serving bowl. Serve immediately.

• •

Nutritional Analysis *(Per Serving)*

313 kcal	29.6 g Carbohydrates
30.6 g Protein	7.2 g Fat

BASIC RECIPE •

Beef and Rice

MAKES 4 SERVINGS			

This recipe should be divided into 4 servings, each containing approximately 357 kcal, or half the daily requirement. To meet your dog's nutritional needs, feed 2 servings a day.

2¼ cups	cooked long-grain brown rice	550 mL
2 cups	drained cooked lean ground beef	500 mL
1⅔ cups	pureed vegetable-and-fruit mix	400 mL
1½ tbsp	canola oil	22 mL
¼ tsp	iodized salt	1 mL
¼ tsp	potassium chloride (salt substitute)	1 mL
	Bonemeal and multivitamin-and-mineral supplements (see Chapter 7, page 200)	

Tips

For basic instructions on how to cook the meats and carbohydrates, see pages 89 to 91.

For information on how to prepare the vegetable-and-fruit mix, see page 88.

For information on additional protein or carbohydrate substitutions, see page 87.

Cubes are ½ inch (1 cm).

The daily caloric requirement of a 25-lb (11.3 kg) dog ranges from 680 to 816 kcal.

1. In a bowl, combine rice, beef, vegetable-and-fruit mix, oil, salt and potassium chloride. Mix thoroughly. Divide into 4 equal portions.

2. Stir supplements into 1 portion and serve immediately. Cover and refrigerate or freeze the remaining portions. Stir supplements into each portion just before serving.

• •

Nutritional Analysis *(Per Serving)*

357 kcal	33.9 g Carbohydrates
19.2 g Protein	15.5 g Fat

Variations

- **Chicken and Rice:** Substitute 3 cups (750 mL) cubed cooked boneless skinless chicken breast for the beef.
- **Turkey and Rice:** Substitute 3 cups (750 mL) cubed cooked boneless skinless turkey breast for the beef.
- **Lamb and Rice:** Substitute 2¼ cups (550 mL) cubed cooked lean boneless lamb for the beef.
- **Meat and Macaroni:** Use the appropriate amount of your preferred meat and substitute 2½ cups (625 mL) drained cooked macaroni for the rice.
- **Meat and Potatoes:** Use the appropriate amount of your preferred meat and substitute 4¼ cups (1.05 L) cubed peeled boiled potatoes for the rice. Omit potassium chloride.

GOURMET RECIPE •

Steak, Eggs and Hash Browns

MAKES 1 SERVING

⅓ cup	cubed (½ inch/1 cm) top sirloin steak	75 mL
1 tsp	canola oil	5 mL
1	large egg, beaten	1
¼ cup	finely chopped tomato	50 mL
3 tbsp	chopped green beans	45 mL
1 tbsp	finely chopped green bell pepper	15 mL
⅛ tsp	minced garlic	0.5 mL
Pinch	dried basil leaves	Pinch
Pinch	iodized salt	Pinch
1 cup	cubed (½ inch/1 cm) peeled boiled potatoes	250 mL
	Bonemeal and multivitamin-and-mineral supplements (see Chapter 7, page 200)	

1. In a nonstick skillet, cook steak over medium heat until no longer pink inside. Transfer to a serving bowl.

2. In same skillet, heat oil over medium heat. Add egg, tomato, green beans, green pepper, garlic, basil and salt. Cook, stirring, for 8 minutes or until vegetables are soft and egg is just set. Let cool until just warm to the touch. Add egg mixture, potatoes and supplements to steak. Mix thoroughly. Serve immediately.

• •

Nutritional Analysis *(Per Serving)*

362 kcal	36.7 g Carbohydrates
23.6 g Protein	13.2 g Fat

Keep Your Eye on the Steak

At one dinner party, Arden of Robert Rose was humiliated when Baron, her 100-lb dog, devoured three momentarily unattended steaks. The four humans shared one steak and a platter of macaroni and cheese. Baron hasn't been invited back.

Lamb Souvlaki in a Pita

MAKES 1 SERVING		
	• *Mini-chopper or immersion blender*	
1¼ tsp	canola oil	6 mL
⅔ cup	cubed (½ inch/1 cm) lean boneless lamb	150 mL
⅛ tsp	dried oregano leaves	0.5 mL
⅛ tsp	minced garlic	0.5 mL
¼ cup	finely chopped tomato	50 mL
2 tbsp	finely chopped peeled cucumber	25 mL
2 tbsp	finely chopped spinach	25 mL
Half	whole wheat pita, torn into bite-size pieces	Half
	Bonemeal and multivitamin-and-mineral supplements (see Chapter 7, page 200)	

1. In a nonstick skillet, heat oil over medium heat. Add lamb, oregano and garlic. Cook, stirring, until lamb is no longer pink inside. Transfer to a serving bowl and let cool until just warm to the touch.

2. In a mini-chopper or using an immersion blender, puree tomato, cucumber and spinach for 1 minute or until smooth. Add to lamb along with pita and supplements. Mix thoroughly. Serve immediately.

• •

Nutritional Analysis *(Per Serving)*

383 kcal	30.6 g Carbohydrates
34.1 g Protein	14.6 g Fat

GOURMET RECIPE •

Spanish Salmon and Rice

MAKES 1 SERVING

1 tsp	canola oil	5 mL
2/3 cup	cubed (1/2 inch/1 cm) boneless skinless salmon	150 mL
1/8 tsp	minced garlic	0.5 mL
1/2 cup	water	125 mL
3 tbsp	finely chopped tomato	45 mL
1 1/2 tbsp	finely chopped zucchini	22 mL
1 tbsp	finely chopped green bell pepper	15 mL
1/8 tsp	dried basil leaves	0.5 mL
Pinch	chili powder	Pinch
Pinch	iodized salt	Pinch
1/4 cup	long-grain brown rice	50 mL
	Bonemeal and multivitamin-and-mineral supplements (see Chapter 7, page 200)	

1. In a saucepan, heat oil over medium heat. Add salmon and garlic. Cook, stirring, until salmon is lightly browned. Add water, tomato, zucchini, green pepper, basil, chili powder and salt. Bring to a boil.

2. Stir in rice. Reduce heat to low. Cover and simmer for 35 minutes or until rice is tender and liquid is absorbed. Remove from heat. Let stand, covered, for 5 minutes. Uncover and let cool until just warm to the touch.

3. Stir in supplements. Transfer to a serving bowl. Serve immediately.

• •

Nutritional Analysis *(Per Serving)*

357 kcal	30.3 g Carbohydrates
26.9 g Protein	13.9 g Fat

30 LBS | *13.6* KG

BASIC RECIPE •

Chicken and Rice

MAKES 4 SERVINGS		

This recipe should be divided into 4 servings, each containing approximately 393 kcal, or half the daily requirement. To meet your dog's nutritional needs, feed 2 servings a day.

3¼ cups	cubed cooked boneless skinless chicken breast	800 mL
2½ cups	cooked long-grain brown rice	625 mL
1⅔ cups	pureed vegetable-and-fruit mix	400 mL
1¾ tbsp	canola oil	23 mL
¼ tsp	iodized salt	1 mL
¼ tsp	potassium chloride (salt substitute)	1 mL
	Bonemeal and multivitamin-and-mineral supplements (see Chapter 7, page 200)	

Tips

For basic instructions on how to cook the meats and carbohydrates, see pages 89 to 91.

For information on how to prepare the vegetable-and-fruit mix, see page 88.

For information on additional protein or carbohydrate substitutions, see page 87.

Cubes are ½ inch (1 cm).

> The daily caloric requirement of a 30-lb (13.6 kg) dog ranges from 779 to 935 kcal.

1. In a bowl, combine chicken, rice, vegetable-and-fruit mix, oil, salt and potassium chloride. Mix thoroughly. Divide into 4 equal portions.

2. Stir supplements into 1 portion and serve immediately. Cover and refrigerate or freeze the remaining portions. Stir supplements into each portion just before serving.

• •

Nutritional Analysis *(Per Serving)*

393 kcal	**37 g Carbohydrates**
37 g Protein	**9.8 g Fat**

Variations

- **Beef and Rice:** Substitute 2¼ cups (550 mL) drained cooked lean ground beef for the chicken.
- **Turkey and Rice:** Substitute 3⅓ cups (825 mL) cubed cooked boneless skinless turkey breast for the chicken.
- **Lamb and Rice:** Substitute 2⅓ cups (575 mL) cubed cooked lean boneless lamb for the chicken.
- **Meat and Macaroni:** Use the appropriate amount of your preferred meat and substitute 2¾ cups (675 mL) drained cooked macaroni for the rice.
- **Meat and Potatoes:** Use the appropriate amount of your preferred meat and substitute 4½ cups (1.125 L) cubed peeled boiled potatoes for the rice. Omit potassium chloride.

GOURMET RECIPE •

Oatmeal, Yogurt and Fruit

MAKES 1 SERVING

Tip

If your dog consumes a milk product without previous exposure to dairy foods, low-level diarrhea may result. To properly break down and digest dairy products, your dog needs an enzyme called lactase, which must be developed gradually. To improve his/her ability to tolerate dairy products, add a small amount of yogurt or cottage cheese to any of the Basic Recipes. After a few weeks, your dog should be able to enjoy the calcium-rich foods from the dairy group and will lap up tasty breakfasts, such as Oatmeal, Yogurt and Fruit.

1 cup	cooked rolled oats	250 mL
3/4 cup	non-fat yogurt	175 mL
1/2 cup	2% cottage cheese	125 mL
1/4 cup	blueberries, thawed if frozen	50 mL
2 tbsp	diced cored apple	25 mL
2 tbsp	chopped peeled banana	25 mL
1 tsp	canola oil	5 mL
1/8 tsp	potassium chloride (salt substitute)	0.5 mL
	Bonemeal and multivitamin-and-mineral supplements (see Chapter 7, page 200)	

1. In a serving bowl, combine oats, yogurt, cottage cheese, blueberries, apple, banana, oil, potassium chloride and supplements. Mix thoroughly. Serve immediately.

• •

Nutritional Analysis *(Per Serving)*

419 kcal	49.4 g Carbohydrates
32.7 g Protein	10.6 g Fat

GOURMET RECIPE •

Chicken Fricassee

MAKES 1 SERVING

Tip
Cubes are ½ inch (1 cm).

1¼ tsp	canola oil	6 mL
¾ cup	cubed boneless skinless chicken breast	175 mL
2 tbsp	cubed chicken livers	25 mL
⅛ tsp	minced garlic	0.5 mL
⅛ tsp	each dried basil and oregano leaves	0.5 mL
Pinch	iodized salt	Pinch
1 cup	water	250 mL
1⅛ cups	cubed peeled potatoes	275 mL
¼ cup	finely chopped zucchini	50 mL
¼ cup	finely chopped tomato	50 mL
1 tbsp	finely chopped green bell pepper	15 mL
½ tsp	fresh lemon juice	2 mL
	Bonemeal and multivitamin-and-mineral supplements (see Chapter 7, page 200)	

1. In a nonstick skillet, heat oil over medium heat. Add chicken, chicken livers, garlic, basil, oregano and salt. Cook, stirring, until chicken is no longer pink inside. Add water and bring to a boil. Add potatoes. Reduce heat, cover and simmer until potatoes are tender.

2. Stir in zucchini, tomato, green pepper and lemon juice. Simmer, stirring occasionally, until vegetables are soft. Let cool until just warm to the touch. Stir in supplements. Transfer to a bowl. Serve immediately.

• •

Nutritional Analysis *(Per Serving)*

399 kcal	**38.7 g Carbohydrates**
39.6 g Protein	**9.1 g Fat**

Greek Dinner
David and Jennifer call this Greek Dinner. Whenever he smells it cooking, their neighbor, Zeus the Doberman, races over.

Stir-Fried Ginger Beef
with Greens

MAKES 1 SERVING

• Wok

1 tsp	canola oil	5 mL
¾ cup	cubed (½ inch/1 cm) top sirloin steak	175 mL
¼ tsp	minced gingerroot	1 mL
⅛ tsp	minced garlic	0.5 mL
¼ cup	chopped green beans, thawed if frozen	50 mL
2 tbsp	green peas, thawed if frozen	25 mL
2 tbsp	finely chopped spinach	25 mL
1½ tsp	light soy sauce	7 mL
⅔ cup	cooked long-grain brown rice	150 mL
Pinch	potassium chloride (salt substitute)	Pinch
	Bonemeal and multivitamin-and-mineral supplements (see Chapter 7, page 200)	

1. In a wok or nonstick skillet, heat oil over medium heat. Add steak, ginger and garlic. Cook, stirring, until steak is no longer pink inside. Add green beans, peas, spinach and soy sauce. Cook, stirring frequently, for 4 minutes or until vegetables are soft. Transfer to a serving bowl.

2. Add rice. Let cool until just warm to the touch. Stir in potassium chloride and supplements. Serve immediately.

• •

Nutritional Analysis *(Per Serving)*

389 kcal	**35.2 g Carbohydrates**
32 g Protein	**12.8 g Fat**

BASIC RECIPE •

Turkey and Rice

MAKES 4 SERVINGS

This recipe should be divided into 4 servings, each containing approximately 444 kcal, or half the daily requirement. To meet your dog's nutritional needs, feed 2 servings a day.

4 cups	cubed cooked boneless skinless turkey breast	1 L
2¾ cups	cooked long-grain brown rice	675 mL
2 cups	pureed vegetable-and-fruit mix	500 mL
1¾ tbsp	canola oil	23 mL
¼ tsp	iodized salt	1 mL
¼ tsp	potassium chloride (salt substitute)	1 mL
	Bonemeal and multivitamin-and-mineral supplements (see Chapter 7, page 201)	

Tips

For basic instructions on how to cook the meats and carbohydrates, see pages 89 to 91.

For information on how to prepare the vegetable-and-fruit mix, see page 88.

For information on additional protein or carbohydrate substitutions, see page 87.

Cubes are ½ inch (1 cm).

The daily caloric requirement of a 35-lb (15.8 kg) dog ranges from 875 to 1,050 kcal.

1. In a bowl, combine turkey, rice, vegetable-and-fruit mix, oil, salt and potassium chloride. Mix thoroughly. Divide into 4 equal portions.

2. Stir supplements into 1 portion and serve immediately. Cover and refrigerate or freeze the remaining portions. Stir supplements into each portion just before serving.

• •

Nutritional Analysis *(Per Serving)*

444 kcal	**41.6 g Carbohydrates**
41.6 g Protein	**10.9 g Fat**

Variations

• **Beef and Rice:** Substitute 2½ cups (625 mL) drained cooked lean ground beef for the turkey.

• **Chicken and Rice:** Substitute 3¾ cups (925 mL) cubed cooked boneless skinless chicken breast for the turkey.

• **Lamb and Rice:** Substitute 2¾ cups (675 mL) cubed cooked lean boneless lamb for the turkey.

• **Meat and Macaroni:** Use the appropriate amount of your preferred meat and substitute 3 cups (750 mL) drained cooked macaroni for the rice.

• **Meat and Potatoes:** Use the appropriate amount of your preferred meat and substitute 5 cups (1.25 L) cubed peeled boiled potatoes for the rice. Omit potassium chloride.

GOURMET RECIPE •

Breakfast Burrito

MAKES 1 SERVING

1¼ tsp	canola oil	6 mL
2 tbsp	finely chopped tomato	25 mL
2 tbsp	corn kernels, thawed if frozen	25 mL
1 tbsp	finely chopped green bell pepper	15 mL
3	large eggs, beaten	3
½ tsp	fresh lime juice	2 mL
¼ tsp	finely chopped cilantro	1 mL
⅛ tsp	each chili powder and minced garlic	0.5 mL
¼ cup	cooked long-grain brown rice	50 mL
Half	10-inch (25 cm) whole wheat tortilla, torn into bite-size pieces	Half
⅛ tsp	potassium chloride (salt substitute)	0.5 mL
	Bonemeal and multivitamin-and-mineral supplements (see Chapter 7, page 201)	

1. In a nonstick skillet, heat oil over medium heat. Add tomato, corn and green pepper. Cook, stirring, until vegetables are soft. Add eggs, lime juice, cilantro, chili powder and garlic. Cook, stirring, until eggs are just set. Add rice and cook, stirring, until liquid is absorbed. Let cool until just warm to the touch.

2. Stir in tortilla, potassium chloride and supplements. Transfer to a serving bowl. Serve immediately.

• •

Nutritional Analysis *(Per Serving)*

459 kcal	**34.6 g Carbohydrates**
22.4 g Protein	**23.7 g Fat**

The Elusive Burrito

One Sunday morning, David and Jennifer prepared a version of this recipe for themselves. As they sat down to eat, they were called outside and left Marley and his cousin T.J. alone in the house. When they returned, their plates had been licked clean and the culprits were looking for more. Hence this recipe.

Luscious Lasagna

MAKES 1 SERVING

Tip

Use a mini-chopper or immersion blender to puree the vegetables, if desired.

- *Preheat oven to 350°F (180°C)*
- *Food processor • 6- by 3-inch (15 by 7.5 cm) mini loaf pan*

1/4 cup	finely chopped tomato	50 mL
2 tbsp	each finely chopped carrot, zucchini and spinach	25 mL
2/3 cup	lean ground beef	150 mL
1/4 cup	water	50 mL
2 tbsp	tomato sauce	25 mL
1/8 tsp	each dried basil and oregano leaves	0.5 mL
1/8 tsp	minced garlic	0.5 mL
1 1/4 tsp	canola oil	6 mL
1 3/4	cooked lasagna noodles, drained	1 3/4
2 tbsp	shredded part-skim mozzarella cheese	25 mL
2 tbsp	part-skim ricotta cheese	25 mL
	Bonemeal and multivitamin-and-mineral supplements (see Chapter 7, page 201)	

1. In a food processor, puree tomato, carrot, zucchini and spinach.

2. In a nonstick skillet over medium heat, cook beef until no longer pink. Drain off fat. Add pureed vegetables, water, tomato sauce, basil, oregano and garlic. Simmer, uncovered, for 10 minutes.

3. Brush pan with oil. Cut half of the noodles to fit bottom of pan. Spread with half of the meat sauce. Sprinkle with half each of the cheeses. Repeat layers. Bake in preheated oven for 30 minutes or until cheese is melted. Let cool until just warm to the touch. Cut into bite-size pieces. Stir in supplements. Transfer to a bowl and serve immediately.

• •

Nutritional Analysis *(Per Serving)*

469 kcal	**40 g Carbohydrates**
30.5 g Protein	**20.5 g Fat**

GOURMET RECIPE •

Divine Dinner Burrito

MAKES 1 SERVING		
1¼ tsp	canola oil	6 mL
⅔ cup	lean ground turkey	150 mL
⅛ tsp	minced garlic	0.5 mL
⅛ tsp	chili powder	0.5 mL
¼ cup	corn kernels, thawed if frozen	50 mL
2 tbsp	finely chopped tomato	25 mL
2 tbsp	tomato sauce	25 mL
1 tbsp	finely chopped green bell pepper	15 mL
½ tsp	chopped cilantro	2 mL
¼ cup	cooked long-grain brown rice	50 mL
Half	10-inch (25 cm) whole wheat tortilla	Half
Pinch	potassium chloride (salt substitute)	Pinch
	Bonemeal and multivitamin-and-mineral supplements (see Chapter 7, page 201)	

1. In a nonstick skillet, heat oil over medium heat. Add turkey, garlic and chili powder. Cook breaking up with a spoon, until no longer pink. Reduce heat to medium-low. Add corn, tomato, tomato sauce and green pepper. Cook, stirring, for 2 minutes or until vegetables are soft. Stir in cilantro and rice. Let cool until just warm to the touch.

2. Spread turkey mixture evenly over tortilla, then roll up. With a sharp knife, cut into ¼-inch (0.5 cm) thick slices.

3. In a serving bowl, combine sliced burrito, potassium chloride and supplements. Mix thoroughly. Serve immediately.

• •

Nutritional Analysis *(Per Serving)*

439 kcal	37.8 g Carbohydrates
27.3 g Protein	19.4 g Fat

BASIC RECIPE •

Lamb and Rice

MAKES 4 SERVINGS

This recipe should be divided into 4 servings, each containing approximately 489 kcal, or half the daily requirement. To meet your dog's nutritional needs, feed 2 servings a day.

3 cups	cubed cooked lean boneless lamb	750 mL
3 cups	cooked long-grain brown rice	750 mL
2 1/4 cups	pureed vegetable-and-fruit mix	550 mL
2 tbsp	canola oil	25 mL
1/2 tsp	iodized salt	2 mL
1/2 tsp	potassium chloride (salt substitute)	2 mL
	Bonemeal and multivitamin-and-mineral supplements (see Chapter 7, page 201)	

1. In a bowl, combine lamb, rice, vegetable-and-fruit mix, oil, salt and potassium chloride. Mix thoroughly. Divide into 4 equal portions.

2. Stir supplements into 1 portion and serve immediately. Cover and refrigerate or freeze the remaining portions. Stir supplements into each portion just before serving.

• •

Tips

For basic instructions on how to cook the meats and carbohydrates, see pages 89 to 91.

For information on how to prepare the vegetable-and-fruit mix, see page 88.

For information on additional protein or carbohydrate substitutions, see page 87.

Cubes are 1/2 inch (1 cm).

The daily caloric requirement of a 40-lb (18.1 kg) dog ranges from 967 to 1,160 kcal.

Nutritional Analysis *(Per Serving)*

489 kcal	45.6 g Carbohydrates
36.4 g Protein	17.6 g Fat

Variations

- **Beef and Rice:** Substitute 2 3/4 cups (675 mL) drained cooked lean ground beef for the lamb.
- **Chicken and Rice:** Substitute 4 cups (1 L) cubed cooked boneless skinless chicken breast for the lamb.
- **Turkey and Rice:** Substitute 4 1/4 cups (1.05 L) cubed cooked boneless skinless turkey breast for the lamb.
- **Meat and Macaroni:** Use the appropriate amount of your preferred meat and substitute 3 1/4 cups (800 mL) drained cooked macaroni for the rice.
- **Meat and Potatoes:** Use the appropriate amount of your preferred meat and substitute 5 1/4 cups (1.3 L) cubed peeled boiled potatoes for the rice. Omit potassium chloride.

GOURMET RECIPE •

Scrambled Eggs with Whole Wheat Toast

MAKES 1 SERVING			
1½ tsp	canola oil		7 mL
¼ cup	finely chopped tomato		50 mL
2 tbsp	finely chopped green bell pepper		25 mL
⅛ tsp	minced garlic		0.5 mL
3	large eggs, beaten		3
2½	slices whole wheat toast, torn into bite-size pieces		2½
Pinch	potassium chloride (salt substitute)		Pinch
	Bonemeal and multivitamin-and-mineral supplements (see Chapter 7, page 201)		

1. In a nonstick skillet, heat oil over medium heat. Add tomato, green pepper and garlic. Cook, stirring, for 5 minutes or until vegetables are soft. Add eggs and cook, stirring, until eggs are just set. Let cool until just warm to the touch.

2. In a serving bowl, combine egg mixture, toast, potassium chloride and supplements. Mix thoroughly. Serve immediately.

• •

Nutritional Analysis *(Per Serving)*

494 kcal	**40.2 g Carbohydrates**
26.1 g Protein	**25 g Fat**

GOURMET RECIPE •

Rotini with Meat Sauce

MAKES 1 SERVING

¾ cup	lean ground beef	175 mL
¼ cup	chopped green beans	50 mL
¼ cup	tomato sauce	50 mL
2 tbsp	finely chopped carrot	25 mL
2 tbsp	finely chopped tomato	25 mL
1 tbsp	finely chopped green bell pepper	15 mL
1 tbsp	finely chopped zucchini	15 mL
1½ tsp	canola oil	7 mL
¼ tsp	dried basil leaves	1 mL
¼ tsp	dried oregano leaves	1 mL
⅛ tsp	minced garlic	0.5 mL
¾ cup	drained cooked rotini	175 mL
	Bonemeal and multivitamin-and-mineral supplements (see Chapter 7, page 201)	

1. In a nonstick skillet over medium heat, cook beef, breaking up with a spoon, until no longer pink. Drain off fat.

2. Reduce heat to low and stir in green beans, tomato sauce, carrot, tomato, green pepper, zucchini, oil, basil, oregano and garlic. Cook, stirring occasionally, for 10 minutes or until vegetables are soft. Stir in rotini. Let cool until just warm to the touch.

3. Stir in supplements. Transfer to a serving bowl. Serve immediately.

• •

Nutritional Analysis *(Per Serving)*

497 kcal	**43.1 g Carbohydrates**
30.9 g Protein	**21.6 g Fat**

Make Mine Italian
Our dogs love this version of pasta in a bolognese sauce.

GOURMET RECIPE •

Chicken Fried Rice

MAKES 1 SERVING

• Wok

1½ tsp	canola oil	7 mL
1 cup	cubed (½ inch/1 cm) boneless skinless chicken breast	250 mL
⅛ tsp	minced garlic	0.5 mL
⅛ tsp	minced gingerroot	0.5 mL
⅓ cup	green peas, thawed if frozen	75 mL
¼ cup	thinly sliced carrot	50 mL
2 tsp	light soy sauce	10 mL
1½ tsp	finely chopped fresh basil leaves	7 mL
¾ cup	cooked long-grain brown rice	175 mL
	Bonemeal and multivitamin-and-mineral supplements (see Chapter 7, page 201)	

1. In a wok or nonstick skillet, heat oil over medium heat. Add chicken, garlic and ginger. Cook, stirring, until chicken is no longer pink inside.

2. Add peas, carrot, soy sauce and basil. Cook, stirring, for 3 minutes or until carrot is tender-crisp. Remove from heat and stir in rice. Let cool until just warm to the touch.

3. Stir in supplements. Transfer to a serving bowl. Serve immediately.

• •

Nutritional Analysis *(Per Serving)*

493 kcal	**46.7 g Carbohydrates**
47.6 g Protein	**11.6 g Fat**

Meals   **125**

BASIC RECIPE •

Beef and Rice

MAKES 4 SERVINGS

This recipe should be divided into 4 servings, each containing approximately 539 kcal, or half the daily requirement. To meet your dog's nutritional needs, feed 2 servings a day.

3¼ cups	cooked long-grain brown rice	800 mL
3 cups	drained cooked lean ground beef	750 mL
2½ cups	pureed vegetable-and-fruit mix	625 mL
2½ tbsp	canola oil	32 mL
½ tsp	iodized salt	2 mL
½ tsp	potassium chloride (salt substitute)	2 mL
	Bonemeal and multivitamin-and-mineral supplements (see Chapter 7, page 202)	

1. In a bowl, combine rice, beef, vegetable-and-fruit mix, oil, salt and potassium chloride. Mix thoroughly. Divide into 4 equal portions.

2. Stir supplements into 1 portion and serve immediately. Cover and refrigerate or freeze the remaining portions. Stir supplements into each portion just before serving.

• •

Tips

For basic instructions on how to cook the meats and carbohydrates, see pages 89 to 91.

For information on how to prepare the vegetable-and-fruit mix, see page 88.

For information on additional protein or carbohydrate substitutions, see page 87.

Cubes are ½ inch (1 cm).

The daily caloric requirement of a 45-lb (20.4 kg) dog ranges from 1,036 to 1,268 kcal.

Nutritional Analysis *(Per Serving)*

539 kcal	**49.7 g Carbohydrates**
28.7 g Protein	**24.3 g Fat**

Variations

- **Chicken and Rice:** Substitute 4½ cups (1.125 L) cubed cooked boneless skinless chicken breast for the beef.
- **Turkey and Rice:** Substitute 4¾ cups (1.175 L) cubed cooked boneless skinless turkey breast for the beef.
- **Lamb and Rice:** Substitute 3¼ cups (800 mL) cubed cooked lean boneless lamb for the beef.
- **Meat and Macaroni:** Use the appropriate amount of your preferred meat and substitute 3½ cups (825 mL) drained cooked macaroni for the rice.
- **Meat and Potatoes:** Use the appropriate amount of your preferred meat and substitute 5¾ cups (1.425 L) cubed peeled boiled potatoes for the rice. Omit potassium chloride.

GOURMET RECIPE •

Steak, Eggs and Hash Browns

MAKES 1 SERVING			
	¾ cup	cubed (½ inch/1 cm) top sirloin steak	175 mL
	1¾ tsp	canola oil	8 mL
	1	large egg, beaten	1
	¼ cup	finely chopped tomato	50 mL
	¼ cup	chopped green beans, thawed if frozen	50 mL
	1 tbsp	finely chopped green bell pepper	15 mL
	⅛ tsp	minced garlic	0.5 mL
	⅛ tsp	dried basil leaves	0.5 mL
	⅛ tsp	iodized salt	0.5 mL
	1½ cups	cubed (½ inch/1 cm) peeled boiled potatoes	375 mL
		Bonemeal and multivitamin-and-mineral supplements (see Chapter 7, page 202)	

1. In a nonstick skillet, cook steak over medium heat until no longer pink inside. Transfer to a serving bowl. Let cool. Wipe skillet clean.

2. In same skillet, heat oil over medium heat. Add egg, tomato, green beans, green pepper, garlic, basil and salt. Cook, stirring, for 8 minutes or until vegetables are soft and egg is just set. Let cool until just warm to the touch.

3. Add egg mixture, potatoes and supplements to steak. Mix thoroughly. Serve immediately.

• •

Nutritional Analysis *(Per Serving)*

549 kcal	**52.4 g Carbohydrates**
38.9 g Protein	**20.3 g Fat**

Texas-Style Chili

MAKES 1 SERVING

¾ cup	lean ground beef	175 mL
¼ cup	corn kernels, thawed if frozen	50 mL
2 tbsp	finely chopped tomato	25 mL
2 tbsp	tomato sauce	25 mL
2 tsp	finely chopped green bell pepper	10 mL
1¾ tsp	canola oil	8 mL
1 tsp	finely chopped cilantro	5 mL
¼ tsp	fresh lime juice	1 mL
⅛ tsp	each chili powder and minced garlic	0.5 mL
¾ cup	cooked long-grain brown rice	175 mL
Pinch	potassium chloride (salt substitute)	Pinch
	Bonemeal and multivitamin-and-mineral supplements (see Chapter 7, page 202)	

1. In a nonstick skillet, cook beef, until no longer pink. Drain off fat. Add corn, tomato, tomato sauce, green pepper, oil, cilantro, lime juice, chili powder and garlic. Cook, stirring occasionally, until vegetables are soft. Let cool.

2. Stir in rice, potassium chloride and supplements. Transfer to a serving bowl. Serve immediately.

• •

Nutritional Analysis *(Per Serving)*

528 kcal	**47.3 g Carbohydrates**
29 g Protein	**24 g Fat**

Please Don't Eat the Tulips

When Jennifer MacKenzie, our recipe editor, saw this chili recipe, she thought of her dog, Daisy. Once, while planting, Jennifer sprinkled tulip bulbs with chili powder to keep pesky squirrels from digging them up. Later, she noticed red powder on Daisy's nose, which smelled suspiciously of chili. Daisy was pleased that Jennifer had seasoned the dirt for her to dig in — and so, it seems, were the squirrels, since tulips pop up in unusual spots around her house every spring.

Beef Stew

MAKES 1 SERVING

2½ tsp	canola oil	12 mL
1 cup	cubed (½ inch/1 cm) top sirloin steak	250 mL
1½ cups	cubed (½ inch/1 cm) peeled potatoes	375 mL
1 cup	water	250 mL
⅛ tsp	dried thyme leaves	0.5 mL
⅛ tsp	minced garlic	0.5 mL
⅛ tsp	iodized salt	0.5 mL
⅓ cup	green peas, thawed if frozen	75 mL
¼ cup	finely chopped carrot	50 mL
2 tbsp	finely chopped celery	25 mL
	Bonemeal and multivitamin-and-mineral supplements (see Chapter 7, page 202)	

1. In a saucepan, heat oil over medium heat. Add steak and cook, stirring, until browned. Add potatoes, water, thyme, garlic and salt. Cover and bring to a boil. Reduce heat, cover and simmer for 10 minutes or until potatoes are almost tender.

2. Stir in peas, carrot and celery. Simmer, uncovered, for 10 minutes or until vegetables are soft. Let cool until just warm to the touch.

3. Stir in supplements. Transfer to a serving bowl. Serve immediately.

• •

Nutritional Analysis *(Per Serving)*

560 kcal	56.2 g Carbohydrates
43.8 g Protein	17.6 g Fat

BASIC RECIPE •

Chicken and Rice

MAKES 4 SERVINGS

This recipe should be divided into 4 servings, each containing approximately 582 kcal, or half the daily requirement. To meet your dog's nutritional needs, feed 2 servings a day.

5 cups	cubed cooked boneless skinless chicken breast	1.25 L
3½ cups	cooked long-grain brown rice	825 mL
2¾ cups	pureed vegetable-and-fruit mix	675 mL
2½ tbsp	canola oil	32 mL
½ tsp	iodized salt	2 mL
½ tsp	potassium chloride (salt substitute)	2 mL
	Bonemeal and multivitamin-and-mineral supplements (see Chapter 7, page 202)	

1. In a bowl, combine chicken, rice, vegetable-and-fruit mix, oil, salt and potassium chloride. Mix thoroughly. Divide into 4 equal portions.

2. Stir supplements into 1 portion and serve immediately. Cover and refrigerate or freeze the remaining portions. Stir supplements into each portion just before serving.

Tips

For basic instructions on how to cook the meats and carbohydrates, see pages 89 to 91.

For information on how to prepare the vegetable-and-fruit mix, see page 88.

For information on additional protein or carbohydrate substitutions, see page 87.

Cubes are ½ inch (1 cm).

The daily caloric requirement of a 50-lb (22.6 kg) dog ranges from 1,143 to 1,372 kcal.

• •

Nutritional Analysis *(Per Serving)*

582 kcal	**53.8 g Carbohydrates**
56.7 g Protein	**14.3 g Fat**

Variations

● **Beef and Rice:** Substitute 3¼ cups (800 mL) drained cooked lean ground beef for the chicken.

● **Turkey and Rice:** Substitute 5 cups (1.25 L) cubed cooked boneless skinless turkey breast for the chicken.

● **Lamb and Rice:** Substitute 3½ cups (825 mL) cubed cooked lean boneless lamb for the chicken.

● **Meat and Macaroni:** Use the appropriate amount of your preferred meat and substitute 4 cups (1 L) drained cooked macaroni for the rice.

● **Meat and Potatoes:** Use the appropriate amount of your preferred meat and substitute 6¼ cups (1.55 L) cubed peeled boiled potatoes for the rice. Omit potassium chloride.

GOURMET RECIPE •

Cottage Cheese, Fruit and Toast

MAKES 1 SERVING		

Tip

If your dog consumes a milk product without previous exposure to dairy foods, low-level diarrhea may result. To properly break down and digest dairy products, your dog needs an enzyme called lactase, which must be developed gradually. To improve his/her ability to tolerate dairy products, add a small amount of yogurt or cottage cheese to any of the Basic Recipes. After a few weeks, your dog should be able to enjoy the calcium-rich foods from the dairy group and will lap up tasty breakfasts, such as Cottage Cheese, Fruit and Toast.

1	large hard-boiled egg, peeled and chopped	1
3	slices whole wheat toast, torn into bite-size pieces	3
¾ cup	2% cottage cheese	175 mL
¼ cup	blueberries, thawed if frozen	50 mL
¼ cup	diced cored apple	50 mL
3 tbsp	chopped peeled banana	45 mL
1¾ tsp	canola oil	8 mL
⅛ tsp	potassium chloride (salt substitute)	0.5 mL
	Bonemeal and multivitamin-and-mineral supplements (see Chapter 7, page 202)	

1. In a serving bowl, combine egg, toast, cottage cheese, blueberries, apple, banana, oil, potassium chloride and supplements. Mix thoroughly. Serve immediately.

• •

Nutritional Analysis *(Per Serving)*

585 kcal	61.2 g Carbohydrates
39.1 g Protein	20.4 g Fat

Dogs and Cheese

We've never known a dog who didn't love cheese — even Maude, who lived with our editor, Judith, and had always been a good little dog until she was led astray by a large wedge of Roquefort. One Halloween evening, Maude trotted into the living room and spotted a cheese tray on the coffee table, ready for guests. Overcome with desire, she acted swiftly. Before anyone could intervene, Maude grabbed the Roquefort and sped to the kitchen, where she swiftly devoured every delicious morsel before anyone could intervene. Fortunately, she didn't appear to suffer any ill effects.

Meals

GOURMET RECIPE •

Red Snapper Stew

MAKES 1 SERVING		
2½ tsp	canola oil	12 mL
1⅓ cups	cubed (½ inch/1 cm) boneless skinless red snapper	325 mL
1¾ cups	cubed (½ inch/1 cm) peeled boiled potatoes	425 mL
¾ cup	water	175 mL
⅓ cup	chopped green beans, thawed if frozen	75 mL
¼ cup	green peas, thawed if frozen	50 mL
2 tbsp	finely chopped carrot	25 mL
⅛ tsp	minced garlic	0.5 mL
⅛ tsp	iodized salt	0.5 mL
Pinch	dried tarragon, thyme or basil leaves	Pinch
	Bonemeal and multivitamin-and-mineral supplements (see Chapter 7, page 202)	

1. In a saucepan, heat oil over medium-low heat. Add snapper and cook, stirring, until lightly browned. Add potatoes, water, green beans, peas, carrot, garlic, salt and tarragon. Cover and cook, stirring occasionally, for 10 minutes or until vegetables are soft. Let cool until just warm to the touch.

2. Stir in supplements. Transfer to a serving bowl. Serve immediately.

• •

Nutritional Analysis *(Per Serving)*

641 kcal	63 g Carbohydrates
61.7 g Protein	15.7 g Fat

GOURMET RECIPE •

Tomato and Chicken Rotini

MAKES 1 SERVING

1¾ tsp	canola oil	8 mL
¾ cup	cubed (½ inch/1 cm) boneless skinless chicken thighs	175 mL
¼ cup	finely chopped tomato	50 mL
¼ cup	finely chopped zucchini	50 mL
3 tbsp	tomato sauce	45 mL
1½ tbsp	finely chopped green bell pepper	22 mL
⅛ tsp	minced garlic	0.5 mL
⅛ tsp	dried basil leaves	0.5 mL
⅛ tsp	dried oregano leaves	0.5 mL
1 cup	drained cooked rotini	250 mL
⅛ tsp	potassium chloride (salt substitute)	0.5 mL
	Bonemeal and multivitamin-and-mineral supplements (see Chapter 7, page 202)	

1. In a saucepan, heat oil over medium heat. Add chicken and cook, stirring, until no longer pink inside. Add tomato, zucchini, tomato sauce, green pepper, garlic, basil and oregano. Cover and cook, stirring occasionally, for 10 minutes or until vegetables are soft.

2. Transfer to a serving bowl. Add rotini and mix thoroughly. Let cool until just warm to the touch. Stir in potassium chloride and supplements. Serve immediately.

• •

Nutritional Analysis *(Per Serving)*

593 kcal	50.6 g Carbohydrates
47 g Protein	19.2 g Fat

BASIC RECIPE •

Lamb and Rice

MAKES 4 SERVINGS

This recipe should be divided into 4 servings, each containing approximately 667 kcal, or half the daily requirement. To meet your dog's nutritional needs, feed 2 servings a day.

4 cups	cubed cooked lean boneless lamb	1 L
4 cups	cooked long-grain brown rice	1 L
3¼ cups	pureed vegetable-and-fruit mix	800 mL
3 tbsp	canola oil	45 mL
½ tsp	iodized salt	2 mL
½ tsp	potassium chloride (salt substitute)	2 mL
	Bonemeal and multivitamin-and-mineral supplements (see Chapter 7, page 203)	

Tips

For basic instructions on how to cook the meats and carbohydrates, see pages 89 to 91.

For information on how to prepare the vegetable-and-fruit mix, see page 88.

For information on additional protein or carbohydrate substitutions, see page 87.

Cubes are ½ inch (1 cm).

1. In a bowl, combine lamb, rice, vegetable-and-fruit mix, oil, salt and potassium chloride. Mix thoroughly. Divide into 4 equal portions.

2. Stir supplements into 1 portion and serve immediately. Cover and refrigerate or freeze the remaining portions. Stir supplements into each portion just before serving.

• •

Nutritional Analysis *(Per Serving)*

667 kcal	**62 g Carbohydrates**
48.6 g Protein	**24.7 g Fat**

The daily caloric requirement of a 60-lb (27.2 kg) dog ranges from 1,310 to 1,573 kcal.

Variations

- **Beef and Rice:** Substitute 3¾ cups (925 mL) drained cooked lean ground beef for the lamb.
- **Chicken and Rice:** Substitute 5½ cups (1.375 L) cubed cooked boneless skinless chicken breast for the lamb.
- **Turkey and Rice:** Substitute 5¾ cups (1.425 L) cubed cooked boneless skinless turkey breast for the lamb.
- **Meat and Macaroni:** Use the appropriate amount of your preferred meat and substitute 4½ cups (1.125 L) drained cooked macaroni for the rice.
- **Meat and Potatoes:** Use the appropriate amount of your preferred meat and substitute 7¼ cups (1.8 L) cubed peeled boiled potatoes for the rice. Omit potassium chloride.

GOURMET RECIPE

Scrambled Eggs with Whole Wheat Toast

MAKES 1 SERVING

2 tsp	canola oil	10 mL
½ cup	finely chopped tomato	125 mL
3 tbsp	finely chopped green bell pepper	45 mL
¼ tsp	minced garlic	1 mL
4	large eggs, beaten	4
3½	slices whole wheat toast, torn into bite-size pieces	3½
⅛ tsp	potassium chloride (salt substitute)	0.5 mL
	Bonemeal and multivitamin-and-mineral supplements (see Chapter 7, page 203)	

1. In a nonstick skillet, heat oil over medium heat. Add tomato, green pepper and garlic. Cook, stirring, for 5 minutes or until vegetables are soft. Add eggs and cook, stirring, until eggs are just set. Let cool until just warm to the touch.

2. In a serving bowl, combine egg mixture, toast, potassium chloride and supplements. Mix thoroughly. Serve immediately.

Nutritional Analysis *(Per Serving)*

680 kcal	58.1 g Carbohydrates
35.7 g Protein	33.5 g Fat

GOURMET RECIPE •

Salmon and Dill Pasta

MAKES 1 SERVING

2 tsp	canola oil	10 mL
1 1/8 cups	cubed (1/2 inch/1 cm) boneless skinless salmon	275 mL
1/3 cup	finely chopped tomato	75 mL
1/3 cup	finely chopped zucchini	75 mL
1/4 cup	finely chopped spinach	50 mL
1/4 tsp	minced garlic	1 mL
1/8 tsp	dried dillweed	0.5 mL
1/8 tsp	iodized salt	0.5 mL
1 1/4 cups	drained cooked rotini or macaroni	300 mL
	Bonemeal and multivitamin-and-mineral supplements (see Chapter 7, page 203)	

1. In a saucepan, heat oil over medium heat. Add salmon and cook, stirring, until fish flakes easily when tested with a fork. Reduce heat to low and add tomato, zucchini, spinach, garlic, dill and salt. Cook, stirring, for 5 minutes or until vegetables are soft. Transfer to a serving bowl. Add rotini and mix thoroughly. Let cool until just warm to the touch. Stir in supplements. Serve immediately.

• •

Nutritional Analysis *(Per Serving)*

682 kcal	**59.1 g Carbohydrates**
53 g Protein	**25.3 g Fat**

A Fishy Story

Although fish may seem like an odd food to feed a dog, many dogs love it. A friend, who recently became converted to the idea of home-prepared diets, regularly cooks gourmet meals featuring swordfish, Arctic char or wild salmon for her elderly standard poodle, who, she was surprised to discover, enjoys fish more than meat. If you're feeding fish to your dog, be sure to remove all the bones.

GOURMET RECIPE •

Lamb Souvlaki in a Pita

MAKES 1 SERVING		

• *Food processor*

1 tbsp	canola oil	15 mL
1 cup	cubed (½ inch/1 cm) lean boneless lamb	250 mL
¼ tsp	dried oregano leaves	1 mL
¼ tsp	minced garlic	1 mL
½ cup	finely chopped tomato	125 mL
¼ cup	finely chopped peeled cucumber	50 mL
¼ cup	finely chopped spinach	50 mL
1	whole wheat pita, torn into bite-size pieces	1
	Bonemeal and multivitamin-and-mineral supplements (see Chapter 7, page 203)	

1. In a nonstick skillet, heat oil over medium heat. Add lamb, oregano and garlic. Cook, stirring, until lamb is no longer pink inside. Transfer to a serving bowl and let cool until just warm to the touch.

2. In a food processor, puree tomato, cucumber and spinach for 1 minute or until smooth. Add to lamb along with pita and supplements. Mix thoroughly. Serve immediately.

• •

Nutritional Analysis *(Per Serving)*

684 kcal	61.3 g Carbohydrates
53.8 g Protein	26.8 g Fat

BASIC RECIPE •

Chicken and Rice

MAKES 4 SERVINGS	6¼ cups	cubed cooked boneless skinless chicken breast	1.55 L
	4½ cups	cooked long-grain brown rice	1.125 L
	3¾ cups	pureed vegetable-and-fruit mix	925 mL
	3 tbsp	canola oil	45 mL
	¾ tsp	iodized salt	4 mL
	¾ tsp	potassium chloride (salt substitute)	4 mL

This recipe should be divided into 4 servings, each containing approximately 737 kcal, or half the daily requirement. To meet your dog's nutritional needs, feed 2 servings a day.

Bonemeal and multivitamin-and-mineral supplements (see Chapter 7, page 203)

1. In a bowl, combine chicken, rice, vegetable-and-fruit mix, oil, salt and potassium chloride. Mix thoroughly. Divide into 4 equal portions.

2. Stir supplements into 1 portion and serve immediately. Cover and refrigerate or freeze the remaining portions. Stir supplements into each portion just before serving.

Tips

For basic instructions on how to cook the meats and carbohydrates, see pages 89 to 91.

For information on how to prepare the vegetable-and-fruit mix, see page 88.

For information on additional protein or carbohydrate substitutions, see page 87.

Cubes are ½ inch (1 cm).

• •

Nutritional Analysis *(Per Serving)*

737 kcal	**70.1 g Carbohydrates**
71.2 g Protein	**17.4 g Fat**

The daily caloric requirement of a 70-lb (31.7 kg) dog ranges from 1,471 to 1,766 kcal.

Variations

● **Beef and Rice:** Substitute 4¼ cups (1.05 L) drained cooked lean ground beef for the chicken.

● **Turkey and Rice:** Substitute 6½ cups (1.625 L) cubed cooked boneless skinless turkey breast for the chicken.

● **Lamb and Rice:** Substitute 4½ cups (1.125 L) cubed cooked lean boneless lamb for the chicken.

● **Meat and Macaroni:** Use the appropriate amount of your preferred meat and substitute 5 cups (1.25 L) drained cooked macaroni for the rice.

● **Meat and Potatoes:** Use the appropriate amount of your preferred meat and substitute 8¼ cups (2.05 L) cubed peeled boiled potatoes for the rice. Omit potassium chloride.

GOURMET RECIPE •

Breakfast Burrito

MAKES 1 SERVING

2¼ tsp	canola oil	11 mL
¼ cup	finely chopped tomato	50 mL
¼ cup	corn kernels, thawed if frozen	50 mL
2 tbsp	finely chopped green bell pepper	25 mL
6	large eggs, beaten	6
½ tsp	finely chopped cilantro	2 mL
½ tsp	fresh lime juice	2 mL
¼ tsp	chili powder	1 mL
¼ tsp	minced garlic	1 mL
½ cup	cooked long-grain brown rice	125 mL
1	10-inch (25 cm) whole wheat tortilla	1
⅛ tsp	potassium chloride (salt substitute)	0.5 mL
	Bonemeal and multivitamin-and-mineral supplements (see Chapter 7, page 203)	

1. In a nonstick skillet, heat oil over medium heat. Add tomato, corn and green pepper. Cook, stirring, for 5 minutes or until vegetables are soft. Add eggs, cilantro, lime juice, chili powder and garlic. Cook, stirring, for 5 minutes or until eggs are just set. Add rice and cook, stirring, until liquid is absorbed. Let cool until just warm to the touch.

2. Spread egg mixture evenly over tortilla, then roll up. With a sharp knife, cut into ¼-inch (0.5 cm) thick slices.

3. In a serving bowl, combine sliced burrito, potassium chloride and supplements. Mix thoroughly. Serve immediately.

• •

Nutritional Analysis *(Per Serving)*

874 kcal	69.8 g Carbohydrates
44.9 g Protein	42.1 g Fat

Basil Chicken and Vegetable Pasta

MAKES 1 SERVING

Tip

If you prefer, substitute 1 tsp (5 mL) dried basil leaves for the fresh basil.

2¼ tsp	canola oil	11 mL
1½ cups	cubed (½ inch/1 cm) boneless skinless chicken breast	375 mL
¼ tsp	minced garlic	1 mL
½ cup	finely chopped tomato	125 mL
½ cup	finely chopped zucchini	125 mL
2 tbsp	finely chopped green bell pepper	25 mL
1½ cups	drained cooked rotini or macaroni	375 mL
1 tbsp	chopped fresh basil leaves	15 mL
¼ tsp	iodized salt	1 mL
½ tsp	freshly grated Parmesan cheese	2 mL
	Bonemeal and multivitamin-and-mineral supplements (see Chapter 7, page 203)	

1. In a nonstick skillet, heat oil over medium heat. Add chicken and garlic. Cook, stirring, until chicken is no longer pink inside. Add tomato, zucchini and green pepper. Cook, stirring, until vegetables are soft. Remove from heat and stir in rotini, basil and salt. Let cool until just warm to the touch. Sprinkle with Parmesan. Stir in supplements. Transfer to a bowl and serve immediately.

• •

Nutritional Analysis *(Per Serving)*

753 kcal	72.7 g Carbohydrates
74 g Protein	16.5 g Fat

A Star Is Born

This recipe saved Dylan's first national TV appearance. Arriving on the set, Dylan concluded that the slippery studio floor bore a striking resemblance to the slippery floors of...ELEVATORS! Dylan decided that he wanted to go home. Fortunately, once he got a whiff of this dish, which was cooking on the set, he faced his fears and conquered the floor.

GOURMET RECIPE •

Chicken Fricassee

MAKES 1 SERVING

2¼ tsp	canola oil	11 mL
1½ cups	cubed (½ inch/1 cm) boneless skinless chicken breast	375 mL
¼ cup	cubed (½ inch/1 cm) chicken livers	50 mL
¼ tsp	minced garlic	1 mL
¼ tsp	dried basil leaves	1 mL
¼ tsp	dried oregano leaves	1 mL
¼ tsp	iodized salt	1 mL
1¾ cups	water	425 mL
2¼ cups	cubed (½ inch/1 cm) peeled potatoes	550 mL
½ cup	finely chopped zucchini	125 mL
½ cup	finely chopped tomato	125 mL
2 tbsp	finely chopped green bell pepper	25 mL
½ tsp	fresh lemon juice	2 mL
	Bonemeal and multivitamin-and-mineral supplements (see Chapter 7, page 203)	

1. In a nonstick skillet, heat oil over medium heat. Add chicken, chicken livers, garlic, basil, oregano and salt. Cook, stirring, until chicken is no longer pink inside. Add water and bring to a boil. Add potatoes. Reduce heat, cover and simmer for 15 minutes or until potatoes are tender.

2. Stir in zucchini, tomato, green pepper and lemon juice. Uncover and simmer, stirring occasionally, for 15 minutes or until vegetables are soft.

3. Let cool until just warm to the touch. Stir in supplements. Transfer to a serving bowl. Serve immediately.

• •

Nutritional Analysis *(Per Serving)*

789 kcal	**77.8 g Carbohydrates**
79.3 g Protein	**17 g Fat**

80 LBS | *36.2* KG

BASIC RECIPE •

Lamb and Rice

MAKES 4 SERVINGS

This recipe should be divided into 4 servings, each containing approximately 824 kcal, or half the daily requirement. To meet your dog's nutritional needs, feed 2 servings a day.

Tips

For basic instructions on how to cook the meats and carbohydrates, see pages 89 to 91.

For information on how to prepare the vegetable-and-fruit mix, see page 88.

For information on additional protein or carbohydrate substitutions, see page 87.

Cubes are $1/2$ inch (1 cm).

The daily caloric requirement of an 80-lb (36.2 kg) dog ranges from 1,626 to 1,951 kcal.

5 cups	cubed cooked lean boneless lamb	1.25 L
5 cups	cooked long-grain brown rice	1.25 L
4 cups	pureed vegetable-and-fruit mix	1 L
3 1/2 tbsp	canola oil	52 mL
3/4 tsp	iodized salt	4 mL
3/4 tsp	potassium chloride (salt substitute)	4 mL
	Bonemeal and multivitamin-and-mineral supplements (see Chapter 7, page 204)	

1. In a bowl, combine lamb, rice, vegetable-and-fruit mix, oil, salt and potassium chloride. Mix thoroughly. Divide into 4 equal portions.

2. Stir supplements into 1 portion and serve immediately. Cover and refrigerate or freeze the remaining portions. Stir supplements into each portion just before serving.

• •

Nutritional Analysis *(Per Serving)*

824 kcal	**77.2 g Carbohydrates**
60.8 g Protein	**29.8 g Fat**

Variations

• **Beef and Rice:** Substitute 4¾ cups (1.175 L) drained cooked lean ground beef for the lamb.

• **Chicken and Rice:** Substitute 7 cups (1.75 L) cubed cooked boneless skinless chicken breast for the lamb.

• **Turkey and Rice:** Substitute 7¼ cups (1.8 L) cubed cooked boneless skinless turkey breast for the lamb.

• **Meat and Macaroni:** Use the appropriate amount of your preferred meat and substitute 5½ cups (1.375 L) drained cooked macaroni for the rice.

• **Meat and Potatoes:** Use the appropriate amount of your preferred meat and substitute 9 cups (2.25 L) cubed peeled boiled potatoes for the rice. Omit potassium chloride.

GOURMET RECIPE •

Oatmeal, Yogurt and Fruit

MAKES 1 SERVING

Tip

If your dog consumes a milk product without previous exposure to dairy foods, low-level diarrhea may result. To properly break down and digest dairy products, your dog needs an enzyme called lactase, which must be developed gradually. To improve his/her ability to tolerate dairy products, add a small amount of yogurt or cottage cheese to any of the Basic Recipes. After a few weeks, your dog should be able to enjoy the calcium-rich foods from the dairy group and will lap up tasty breakfasts, such as Oatmeal, Yogurt and Fruit.

2 cups	cooked rolled oats	500 mL
1½ cups	non-fat yogurt	375 mL
¾ cup	2% cottage cheese	175 mL
½ cup	blueberries, thawed if frozen	125 mL
¼ cup	diced cored apple	50 mL
¼ cup	chopped peeled banana	50 mL
2¾ tsp	canola oil	14 mL
¼ tsp	potassium chloride (salt substitute)	1 mL
	Bonemeal and multivitamin-and-mineral supplements (see Chapter 7, page 204)	

1. In a serving bowl, combine oats, yogurt, cottage cheese, blueberries, apple, banana, oil, potassium chloride and supplements. Mix thoroughly. Serve immediately.

• •

Nutritional Analysis *(Per Serving)*

820 kcal	**97.4 g Carbohydrates**
57.7 g Protein	**24.1 g Fat**

Hot Weather Food
Our dogs really enjoy this for breakfast. It's especially refreshing in the heat of the summer months.

GOURMET RECIPE •

Divine Dinner Burrito

MAKES 1 SERVING

2½ tsp	canola oil	12 mL
1¼ cups	lean ground turkey	300 mL
¼ tsp	minced garlic	1 mL
¼ tsp	chili powder	1 mL
½ cup	corn kernels, thawed if frozen	125 mL
¼ cup	finely chopped tomato	50 mL
¼ cup	tomato sauce	50 mL
2 tbsp	finely chopped green bell pepper	25 mL
1 tsp	finely chopped cilantro	5 mL
½ cup	cooked long-grain brown rice	125 mL
1	10-inch (25 cm) whole wheat tortilla	1
⅛ tsp	potassium chloride (salt substitute)	0.5 mL
	Bonemeal and multivitamin-and-mineral supplements (see Chapter 7, page 204)	

1. In a nonstick skillet, heat oil over medium heat. Add turkey, garlic and chili powder. Cook, breaking up with a spoon, until no longer pink. Reduce heat to medium-low. Add corn, tomato, tomato sauce and green pepper. Cook, stirring, for 2 minutes or until vegetables are soft. Stir in cilantro and rice. Let cool until just warm to the touch.

2. Spread turkey mixture evenly over tortilla, then roll up. With a sharp knife, cut into ¼-inch (0.5 cm) thick slices.

3. In a serving bowl, combine sliced burrito, potassium chloride and supplements. Mix thoroughly. Serve immediately.

• •

Nutritional Analysis *(Per Serving)*

879 kcal	**75.7 g Carbohydrates**
54.8 g Protein	**38.9 g Fat**

GOURMET RECIPE

Rotini with Meat Sauce

MAKES 1 SERVING			
8 oz	lean ground beef	250 g
½ cup	chopped green beans, thawed if frozen	125 mL
½ cup	tomato sauce	125 mL
¼ cup	finely chopped carrot	50 mL
¼ cup	finely chopped tomato	50 mL
2 tbsp	finely chopped green bell pepper	25 mL
2 tbsp	finely chopped zucchini	25 mL
2½ tsp	canola oil	12 mL
½ tsp	dried basil leaves	2 mL
½ tsp	dried oregano leaves	2 mL
¼ tsp	minced garlic	1 mL
1⅓ cups	drained cooked rotini	325 mL
	Bonemeal and multivitamin-and-mineral supplements (see Chapter 7, page 204)	

1. In a nonstick skillet over medium heat, cook beef, breaking up with a spoon, until no longer pink. Drain off fat.

2. Reduce heat to low and stir in green beans, tomato sauce, carrot, tomato, green pepper, zucchini, oil, basil, oregano and garlic. Cook, stirring occasionally, for 10 minutes or until vegetables are soft. Stir in rotini. Let cool until just warm to the touch.

3. Stir in supplements. Transfer to a serving bowl. Serve immediately.

Nutritional Analysis *(Per Serving)*

869 kcal	81.1 g Carbohydrates
53 g Protein	36.1 g Fat

BASIC RECIPE •

Chicken and Rice

MAKES 4 SERVINGS			

This recipe should be divided into 4 servings, each containing approximately 888 kcal, or half the daily requirement. To meet your dog's nutritional needs, feed 2 servings a day.

7¾ cups	cubed cooked boneless skinless chicken breast	1.925 L
5¼ cups	cooked long-grain brown rice	1.3 L
4¾ cups	pureed vegetable-and-fruit mix	1.175 L
3½ tbsp	canola oil	52 mL
¾ tsp	iodized salt	4 mL
¾ tsp	potassium chloride (salt substitute)	4 mL
	Bonemeal and multivitamin-and-mineral supplements (see Chapter 7, page 204)	

Tips

For basic instructions on how to cook the meats and carbohydrates, see pages 89 to 91.

For information on how to prepare the vegetable-and-fruit mix, see page 88.

For information on additional protein or carbohydrate substitutions, see page 87.

Cubes are ½ inch (1 cm).

The daily caloric requirement of a 90-lb (40.8 kg) dog ranges from 1,776 to 2,132 kcal.

1. In a bowl, combine chicken, rice, vegetable-and-fruit mix, oil, salt and potassium chloride. Mix thoroughly. Divide into 4 equal portions.

2. Stir supplements into 1 portion and serve immediately. Cover and refrigerate or freeze the remaining portions. Stir supplements into each portion just before serving.

• •

Nutritional Analysis *(Per Serving)*

888 kcal	83.4 g Carbohydrates
87.9 g Protein	20.5 g Fat

Variations

● **Beef and Rice:** Substitute 5¼ cups (1.3 L) drained cooked lean ground beef for the chicken.

● **Turkey and Rice:** Substitute 8 cups (2 L) cubed cooked boneless skinless turkey breast for the chicken.

● **Lamb and Rice:** Substitute 5½ cups (1.375 L) cubed cooked lean boneless lamb for the chicken.

● **Meat and Macaroni:** Use the appropriate amount of your preferred meat and substitute 6 cups (1.5 L) drained cooked macaroni for the rice.

● **Meat and Potatoes:** Use the appropriate amount of your preferred meat and substitute 9½ cups (2.375 L) cubed peeled boiled potatoes for the rice. Omit potassium chloride.

GOURMET RECIPE •

Cottage Cheese, Fruit and Toast

MAKES 1 SERVING

Tip

If your dog consumes a milk product without previous exposure to dairy foods, low-level diarrhea may result. To properly break down and digest dairy products, your dog needs an enzyme called lactase, which must be developed gradually. To improve his/her ability to tolerate dairy products, add a small amount of yogurt or cottage cheese to any of the Basic Recipes. After a few weeks, your dog should be able to enjoy the calcium-rich foods from the dairy group and will lap up tasty breakfasts, such as Cottage Cheese, Fruit and Toast.

2	large hard-boiled eggs, peeled and chopped	2
4½	slices whole wheat toast, torn into bite-size pieces	4½
1 cup	2% cottage cheese	250 mL
½ cup	blueberries, thawed if frozen	125 mL
¼ cup	diced cored apple	50 mL
¼ cup	chopped peeled banana	50 mL
1 tbsp	canola oil	15 mL
⅛ tsp	potassium chloride (salt substitute)	0.5 mL
	Bonemeal and multivitamin-and-mineral supplements (see Chapter 7, page 204)	

1. In a serving bowl, combine egg, toast, cottage cheese, blueberries, apple, banana, oil, potassium chloride and supplements. Mix thoroughly. Serve immediately.

• •

Nutritional Analysis *(Per Serving)*

904 kcal	90.6 g Carbohydrates
57.7 g Protein	34.7 g Fat

GOURMET RECIPE •

Luscious Lasagna

MAKES 1 SERVING

Tip
Use a mini-chopper or immersion blender to puree the vegetables, if desired.

• *Preheat oven to 350°F (180°C)*
• *Food processor • 8½- by 4½-inch (1.5 L) loaf pan*

½ cup	finely chopped tomato	125 mL
¼ cup	each finely chopped carrots, zucchini and spinach	50 mL
1 cup	lean ground beef	250 mL
¼ cup	water	50 mL
¼ cup	tomato sauce	50 mL
¼ tsp	each dried basil and oregano leaves	1 mL
¼ tsp	minced garlic	1 mL
1 tbsp	canola oil	15 mL
3½	cooked lasagna noodles, drained	3½
¼ cup	shredded part-skim mozzarella cheese	50 mL
¼ cup	part-skim ricotta cheese	50 mL
	Bonemeal and multivitamin-and-mineral supplements (see Chapter 7, page 204)	

1. In a food processor, puree tomato, carrot, zucchini and spinach.

2. In a nonstick skillet over medium heat, cook beef until no longer pink.. Drain off fat. Add pureed vegetables, water, tomato sauce, basil, oregano and garlic. Simmer, uncovered, for 10 minutes.

3. Brush pan with oil. Cut half of the noodles to fit bottom of pan. Spread with half of the meat sauce. Sprinkle with half each of the cheeses. Repeat layers. Bake in preheated oven for 30 minutes or until cheese is melted. Let cool until just warm to the touch. Cut into bite-size pieces. Stir in supplements. Transfer to a serving bowl and serve immediately.

• •

Nutritional Analysis *(Per Serving)*

892 kcal	**81.8 g Carbohydrates**
53 g Protein	**38.8 g Fat**

GOURMET RECIPE •

Stir-Fried Ginger Beef with Greens

MAKES 1 SERVING

• Wok

1 tbsp	canola oil	15 mL
2 cups	cubed (½ inch/1 cm) top sirloin steak	500 mL
½ tsp	minced gingerroot	2 mL
¼ tsp	minced garlic	1 mL
½ cup	chopped green beans	125 mL
¼ cup	green peas	50 mL
¼ cup	finely chopped spinach	50 mL
1 tbsp	light soy sauce	15 mL
1¼ cups	cooked long-grain brown rice	300 mL
⅛ tsp	potassium chloride (salt substitute)	0.5 mL
	Bonemeal and multivitamin-and-mineral supplements (see Chapter 7, page 204)	

1. In a nonstick skillet, heat oil over medium heat. Add steak, ginger and garlic. Cook, stirring, until steak is no longer pink inside. Add beans, peas, spinach and soy sauce. Cook, stirring frequently, for 4 minutes or until vegetables are soft. Transfer to a bowl. Add rice. Let cool until just warm to the touch. Stir in potassium chloride and supplements. Serve immediately.

• •

Nutritional Analysis *(Per Serving)*

932 kcal	71.5 g Carbohydrates
82.5 g Protein	34 g Fat

Party Food
Although lasagna (see opposite page) is a bit complicated to make, it is a favorite at David and Jennifer's house and is usually expected fare at the many birthday celebrations.

BASIC RECIPE •

Lamb and Rice

MAKES 4 SERVINGS

This recipe should be divided into 4 servings, each containing approximately 977 kcal, or half the daily requirement. To meet your dog's nutritional needs, feed 2 servings a day.

6 cups	cubed cooked lean boneless lamb	1.5 L
5¾ cups	cooked long-grain brown rice	1.425 L
5¼ cups	pureed vegetable-and-fruit mix	1.3 L
¼ cup	canola oil	50 mL
1 tsp	iodized salt	5 mL
1 tsp	potassium chloride (salt substitute)	5 mL
	Bonemeal and multivitamin-and-mineral supplements (see Chapter 7, page 205)	

1. In a bowl, combine lamb, rice, vegetable-and-fruit mix, oil, salt and potassium chloride. Mix thoroughly. Divide into 4 equal portions.

2. Stir supplements into 1 portion and serve immediately. Cover and refrigerate or freeze the remaining portions. Stir supplements into each portion just before serving.

• •

Nutritional Analysis *(Per Serving)*

977 kcal	91.6 g Carbohydrates
72.9 g Protein	35 g Fat

Tips

For basic instructions on how to cook the meats and carbohydrates, see pages 89 to 91.

For information on how to prepare the vegetable-and-fruit mix, see page 88.

For information on additional protein or carbohydrate substitutions, see page 87.

Cubes are ½ inch (1 cm).

The daily caloric requirement of a 100-lb (45.3 kg) dog ranges from 1,922 to 2,307 kcal.

Variations

- **Beef and Rice:** Substitute 5½ cups (1.375 L) drained cooked lean ground beef for the lamb.
- **Chicken and Rice:** Substitute 8¼ cups (2.05 L) cubed cooked boneless skinless chicken breast for the lamb.
- **Turkey and Rice:** Substitute 8½ cups (2.125 L) cubed cooked boneless skinless turkey breast for the lamb.
- **Meat and Macaroni:** Use the appropriate amount of your preferred meat and substitute 6½ cups (1.625 L) drained cooked macaroni for the rice.
- **Meat and Potatoes:** Use the appropriate amount of your preferred meat and substitute 10½ cups (2.625 L) cubed peeled boiled potatoes for the rice. Omit potassium chloride.

GOURMET RECIPE •

Steak, Eggs and Hash Browns

MAKES 1 SERVING			
1½ cups	cubed (½ inch/1 cm) top sirloin steak	375 mL
1½ tbsp	canola oil	22 mL
2	large eggs, beaten	2
½ cup	finely chopped tomato	125 mL
½ cup	chopped green beans, thawed if frozen	125 mL
2 tbsp	finely chopped green bell pepper	25 mL
¼ tsp	each minced garlic, dried basil leaves and iodized salt	1 mL
2½ cups	cubed (½ inch/1 cm) peeled boiled potatoes	625 mL
	Bonemeal and multivitamin-and-mineral supplements (see Chapter 7, page 205)	

1. In a nonstick skillet, cook steak over medium heat until no longer pink inside. Transfer to a serving bowl. Let cool. Wipe skillet clean. In same skillet, heat oil over medium heat. Add eggs, tomato, green beans, green pepper, garlic, basil and salt. Cook, stirring, for 8 minutes or until vegetables are soft and eggs are just set. Let cool until just warm to the touch.

2. Add egg mixture, potatoes and supplements to steak. Mix thoroughly. Serve immediately.

• •

Nutritional Analysis *(Per Serving)*

1,071 kcal	89.7 g Carbohydrates
76 g Protein	45 g Fat

Sunday Brunch
David and Jennifer particularly enjoy weekends, because they get to hang out with their dogs all day. All five enjoy this tasty breakfast so much that it has become a Sunday morning staple!

GOURMET RECIPE •

Spanish Salmon and Rice

MAKES 1 SERVING

1 tbsp	canola oil	15 mL
1¾ cups	cubed (½ inch/1 cm) boneless skinless salmon	425 mL
¼ tsp	minced garlic	1 mL
1 cup	water	250 mL
½ cup	finely chopped tomato	125 mL
¼ cup	finely chopped zucchini	50 mL
2 tbsp	finely chopped green bell pepper	25 mL
¼ tsp	dried basil leaves	1 mL
¼ tsp	chili powder	1 mL
⅛ tsp	iodized salt	0.5 mL
½ cup	long-grain brown rice	125 mL
	Bonemeal and multivitamin-and-mineral supplements (see Chapter 7, page 205)	

1. In a saucepan, heat oil over medium heat. Add salmon and garlic. Cook, stirring, until salmon is lightly browned. Add water, tomato, zucchini, green pepper, basil, chili powder and salt. Bring to a boil.

2. Stir in rice. Reduce heat to low. Cover and simmer for 35 minutes or until rice is tender and liquid is absorbed. Remove from heat. Let stand, covered, for 5 minutes. Uncover and let cool until just warm to the touch.

3. Stir in supplements. Transfer a to serving bowl. Serve immediately.

• •

Nutritional Analysis *(Per Serving)*

980 kcal	80.9 g Carbohydrates
74.7 g Protein	38.8 g Fat

GOURMET RECIPE •

Barbecued Hamburgers

MAKES 1 SERVING

• *Preheat barbecue*

1¾ cups	lean ground beef	425 mL
3	whole wheat hamburger buns	3
¾ cup	finely chopped tomato	175 mL
¾ cup	finely chopped lettuce	175 mL
1 tbsp	canola oil	15 mL
⅛ tsp	potassium chloride (salt substitute)	0.5 mL
	Bonemeal and multivitamin-and-mineral supplements (see Chapter 7, page 205)	

1. Form beef into three ½-inch (1 cm) thick patties. Place on preheated barbecue and grill, turning once, until no longer pink inside. Let cool until just warm to the touch.

2. Cut burgers and buns into bite-size pieces. In a serving bowl, combine burgers, buns, tomato, lettuce, oil, potassium chloride and supplements. Mix thoroughly. Serve immediately.

• •

Nutritional Analysis *(Per Serving)*

1,093 kcal	87.1 g Carbohydrates
74.2 g Protein	51 g Fat

BASIC RECIPE •

Beef and Rice

MAKES 4 SERVINGS		
6 cups	drained cooked lean ground beef	1.5 L
6 cups	cooked long-grain brown rice	1.5 L
6 cups	pureed vegetable-and-fruit mix	1.5 L
¼ cup	canola oil	50 mL
1 tsp	iodized salt	5 mL
1 tsp	potassium chloride (salt substitute)	5 mL
	Bonemeal and multivitamin-and-mineral supplements (see Chapter 7, page 205)	

This recipe should be divided into 4 servings, each containing approximately 1,034 kcal, or half the daily requirement. To meet your dog's nutritional needs, feed 2 servings a day.

1. In a bowl, combine beef, rice, vegetable-and-fruit mix, oil, salt and potassium chloride. Mix thoroughly. Divide into 4 equal portions.

2. Stir supplements into 1 portion and serve immediately. Cover and refrigerate or freeze the remaining portions. Stir supplements into each portion just before serving.

Tips

For basic instructions on how to cook the meats and carbohydrates, see pages 89 to 91.

For information on how to prepare the vegetable-and-fruit mix, see page 88.

For information on additional protein or carbohydrate substitutions, see page 87.

Cubes are ½ inch (1 cm).

• •

Nutritional Analysis *(Per Serving)*

1,034 kcal	97.8 g Carbohydrates
57.3 g Protein	44.7 g Fat

Variations

- **Chicken and Rice:** Substitute 8¾ cups (2.175 L) cubed cooked boneless skinless chicken breast for the beef.
- **Turkey and Rice:** Substitute 9¼ cups (2.3 L) cubed cooked boneless skinless turkey breast for the beef.
- **Lamb and Rice:** Substitute 6¼ cups (1.55 L) cubed cooked lean boneless lamb for the beef.
- **Meat and Macaroni:** Use the appropriate amount of your preferred meat and substitute 6¾ cups (1.675 L) drained cooked macaroni for the rice.
- **Meat and Potatoes:** Use the appropriate amount of your preferred meat and substitute 11 cups (2.75 L) cubed peeled boiled potatoes for the rice. Omit potassium chloride.

The daily caloric requirement of a 110-lb (49.8 kg) dog ranges from 2,065 to 2,478 kcal.

GOURMET RECIPE •

Oatmeal, Yogurt and Fruit

MAKES 1 SERVING

2 1/2 cups	cooked rolled oats	625 mL
2 cups	non-fat yogurt	500 mL
1 cup	2% cottage cheese	250 mL
2/3 cup	blueberries, thawed if frozen	150 mL
1/3 cup	diced cored apple	75 mL
1/3 cup	chopped peeled banana	75 mL
1 1/2 tbsp	canola oil	22 mL
1/4 tsp	potassium chloride (salt substitute)	1 mL
	Bonemeal and multivitamin-and-mineral supplements (see Chapter 7, page 205)	

Tip

If your dog consumes a milk product without previous exposure to dairy foods, low-level diarrhea may result. To properly break down and digest dairy products, your dog needs an enzyme called lactase, which must be developed gradually. To improve his/her ability to tolerate dairy products, add a small amount of yogurt or cottage cheese to any of the Basic Recipes. After a few weeks, your dog should be able to enjoy the calcium-rich foods from the dairy group and will lap up tasty breakfasts, such as Oatmeal, Yogurt and Fruit.

1. In a serving bowl, combine oats, yogurt, cottage cheese, blueberries, apple, banana, oil, potassium chloride and supplements. Mix thoroughly. Serve immediately.

• •

Nutritional Analysis *(Per Serving)*

1,103 kcal	126.2 g Carbohydrates
75.9 g Protein	35.2 g Fat

GOURMET RECIPE •

Chicken Fried Rice

MAKES 1 SERVING

• Wok

1 tbsp	canola oil	15 mL
2 cups	cubed (½ inch/1 cm) boneless skinless chicken breast	500 mL
¼ tsp	minced garlic	1 mL
¼ tsp	minced gingerroot	1 mL
¾ cup	green peas, thawed if frozen	175 mL
½ cup	finely chopped carrot	125 mL
1 tbsp	light soy sauce	15 mL
1 tbsp	chopped fresh basil leaves (or 1 tsp/5 mL dried basil leaves)	15 mL
1¾ cups	cooked long-grain brown rice	425 mL
	Bonemeal and multivitamin-and-mineral supplements (see Chapter 7, page 205)	

1. In a wok or nonstick skillet, heat oil over medium heat. Add chicken, garlic and ginger. Cook, stirring, until chicken is no longer pink inside.

2. Add peas, carrot, soy sauce and basil. Cook, stirring, for 3 minutes or until carrot is tender-crisp. Remove from heat and stir in rice. Let cool until just warm to the touch. Stir in supplements. Transfer to a serving bowl. Serve immediately.

• •

Nutritional Analysis *(Per Serving)*

1,048 kcal	106 g Carbohydrates
96.5 g Protein	23.9 g Fat

GOURMET RECIPE

Beef Stew

MAKES 1 SERVING

1 ½ tbsp	canola oil	22 mL
2 cups	cubed (½ inch/1 cm) top sirloin steak	500 mL
2 ½ cups	cubed (½ inch/1 cm) peeled potatoes	625 mL
2 cups	water	500 mL
¼ tsp	each dried thyme leaves, minced garlic and iodized salt	1 mL
¾ cup	green peas, thawed if frozen	175 mL
½ cup	finely chopped carrot	125 mL
¼ cup	finely chopped celery	50 mL
	Bonemeal and multivitamin-and-mineral supplements (see Chapter 7, page 205)	

1. In a large saucepan, heat oil over medium heat. Add steak and cook, stirring, until browned. Add potatoes, water, thyme, garlic and salt. Cover and bring to a boil. Reduce heat and simmer until potatoes are almost tender.

2. Stir in peas, carrot and celery. Uncover and simmer for 10 minutes or until vegetables are soft. Let cool until just warm to the touch. Stir in supplements. Transfer to a serving bowl. Serve immediately.

Nutritional Analysis *(Per Serving)*

1,098 kcal	98 g Carbohydrates
86.3 g Protein	39.7 g Fat

No More Chasing Cows

Harris' affinity for beef is the main reason he ended up at the animal shelter – he spent too much time chasing the neighbor's cows. Guess his former humans hadn't heard of a fence. Now, living with David and Jennifer and enjoying his large fenced yard, Harris' fondness for beef is satisfied by delicious meals like this.

BASIC RECIPE •

Chicken and Rice

MAKES 4 SERVINGS		

This recipe should be divided into 4 servings, each containing approximately 1,124 kcal, or half the daily requirement. To meet your dog's nutritional needs, feed 2 servings a day.

9½ cups	cubed cooked boneless skinless chicken breast	2.375 L
6½ cups	cooked long-grain brown rice	1.625 L
6¼ cups	pureed vegetable-and-fruit mix	1.55 L
5 tbsp	canola oil	70 mL
1 tsp	iodized salt	5 mL
1 tsp	potassium chloride (salt substitute)	5 mL
	Bonemeal and multivitamin-and-mineral supplements (see Chapter 7, page 206)	

Tips

For basic instructions on how to cook the meats and carbohydrates, see pages 89 to 91.

For information on how to prepare the vegetable-and-fruit mix, see page 88.

For information on additional protein or carbohydrate substitutions, see page 87.

Cubes are ½ inch (1cm).

1. In a bowl, combine chicken, rice, vegetable-and-fruit mix, oil, salt and potassium chloride. Mix thoroughly. Divide into 4 equal portions.

2. Stir supplements into 1 portion and serve immediately. Cover and refrigerate or freeze the remaining portions. Stir supplements into each portion just before serving.

• •

Nutritional Analysis *(Per Serving)*

1,124 kcal		**104.9 g Carbohydrates**
108.1 g Protein		**28 g Fat**

The daily caloric requirement of a 120-lb (54.4 kg) dog ranges from 2,204 to 2,645 kcal.

Variations

- **Beef and Rice:** Substitute 6¼ cups (1.55 L) drained cooked lean ground beef for the chicken.
- **Lamb and Rice:** Substitute 6¾ cups (1.675 L) cubed cooked lean boneless lamb for the chicken.
- **Turkey and Rice:** Substitute 10 cups (2.5 L) cubed cooked boneless skinless turkey breast for the chicken.
- **Meat and Macaroni:** Use the appropriate amount of your preferred meat and substitute 7¼ cups (1.8 L) drained cooked macaroni for the rice.
- **Meat and Potatoes:** Use the appropriate amount of your preferred meat and substitute 12 cups (3 L) cubed peeled boiled potatoes for the rice. Omit potassium chloride.

GOURMET RECIPE •

Steak, Eggs and Hash Browns

MAKES 1 SERVING			
1¾ cups	cubed (½ inch/1 cm) top sirloin steak	425 mL
1½ tbsp	canola oil	22 mL
2	large eggs, beaten	2
¾ cup	chopped green beans, thawed if frozen	175 mL
⅔ cup	finely chopped tomato	150 mL
2 tbsp	finely chopped green bell pepper	25 mL
½ tsp	minced garlic	2 mL
½ tsp	dried basil leaves	2 mL
¼ tsp	iodized salt	1 mL
3 cups	cubed (½ inch/1 cm) peeled boiled potatoes	750 mL
	Bonemeal and multivitamin-and-mineral supplements (see Chapter 7, page 206)	

1. In a nonstick skillet, cook steak over medium heat until no longer pink inside. Transfer to a serving bowl. Let cool. Wipe skillet clean.

2. In same skillet, heat oil over medium heat. Add eggs, green beans, tomato, green pepper, garlic, basil and salt. Cook, stirring, for 8 minutes or until vegetables are soft and eggs are just set. Let cool until just warm to the touch.

3. Add egg mixture, potatoes and supplements to steak. Mix thoroughly. Serve immediately.

• •

Nutritional Analysis *(Per Serving)*

1,205 kcal	107.2 g Carbohydrates
87.3 g Protein	47.2 g Fat

GOURMET RECIPE •

Texas-Style Chili

MAKES 1 SERVING

1¾ cups	lean ground beef	425 mL
¼ cup	finely chopped tomato	50 mL
⅓ cup	each corn kernels and tomato sauce	75 mL
1 tbsp	finely chopped green bell pepper	15 mL
1 tbsp	finely chopped cilantro	15 mL
1 tbsp	canola oil	15 mL
½ tsp	each chili powder, minced garlic and fresh lime juice	2 mL
1½ cups	cooked long-grain brown rice	375 mL
¼ tsp	potassium chloride (salt substitute)	1 mL
	Bonemeal and multivitamin-and-mineral supplements (see Chapter 7, page 206)	

1. In a nonstick skillet over medium heat, cook beef, until no longer pink. Drain off fat. Add tomato, corn, tomato sauce, green pepper, cilantro, oil, chili powder, garlic and lime juice. Cook, stirring occasionally, for 10 minutes or until vegetables are soft. Add rice. Let cool until just warm to the touch. Stir in potassium chloride and supplements. Transfer to a serving bowl. Serve immediately.

• •

Nutritional Analysis *(Per Serving)*

1,103 kcal	93.5 g Carbohydrates
65.8 g Protein	49.7 g Fat

Comfort Food

When David and Jennifer adopted Marley, he was 18 months old and had lived in five different homes. After his first night, they drove him to the veterinarian for an exam. David could see Marley looking in the rearview mirror apparently asking, "Why are you taking me back? What did I do wrong?" Then he lay down and turned his head away. No consoling worked. He didn't perk up until they arrived home and had this chili for dinner. Marley still gets excited when he smells it cooking. Maybe it's his version of comfort food.

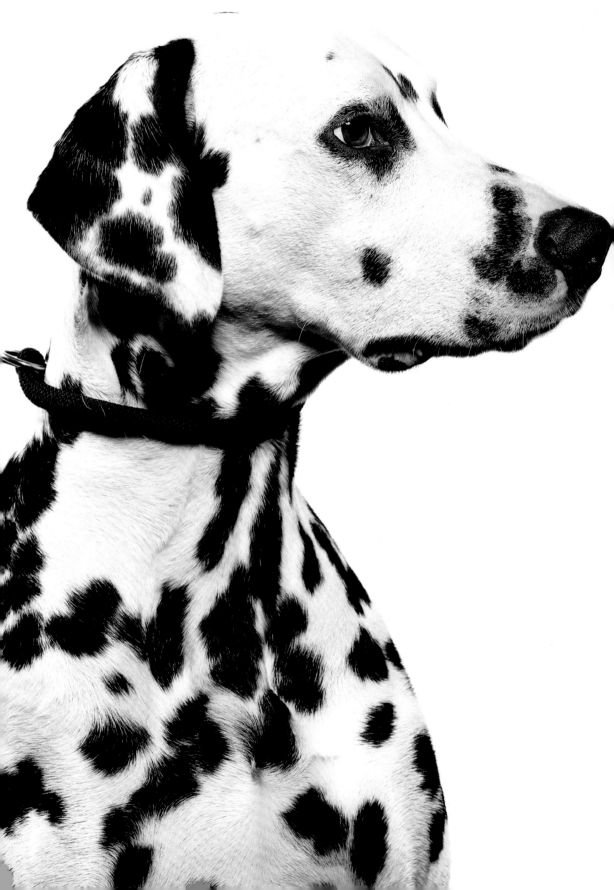

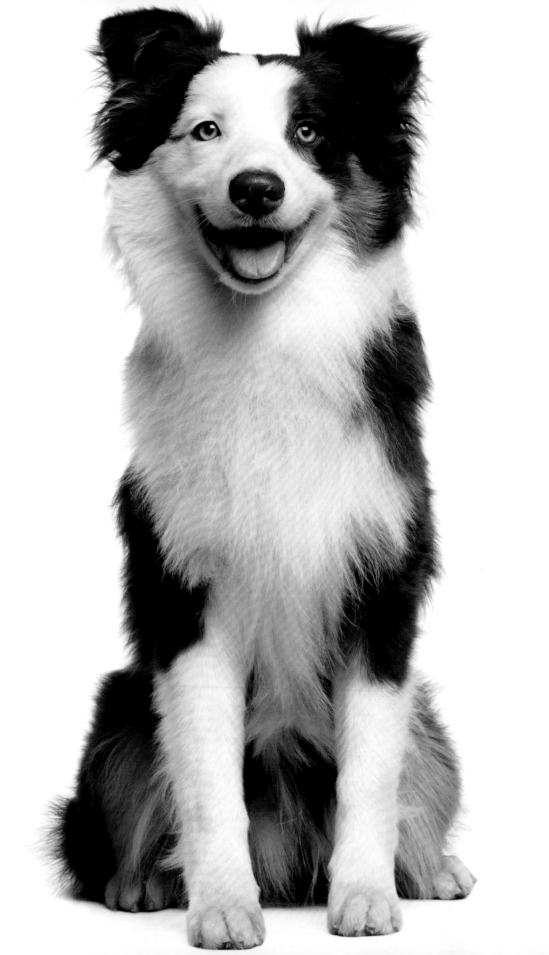

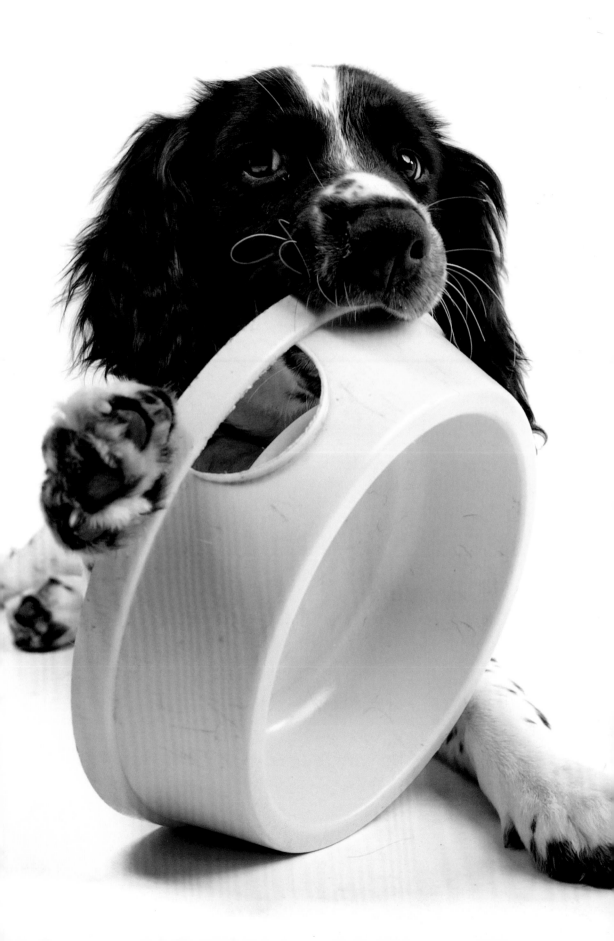

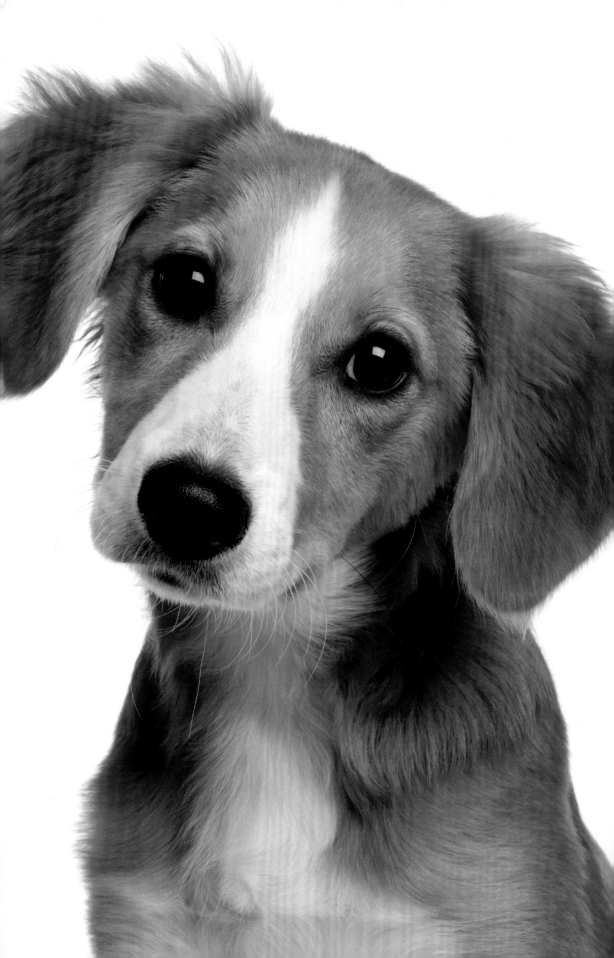

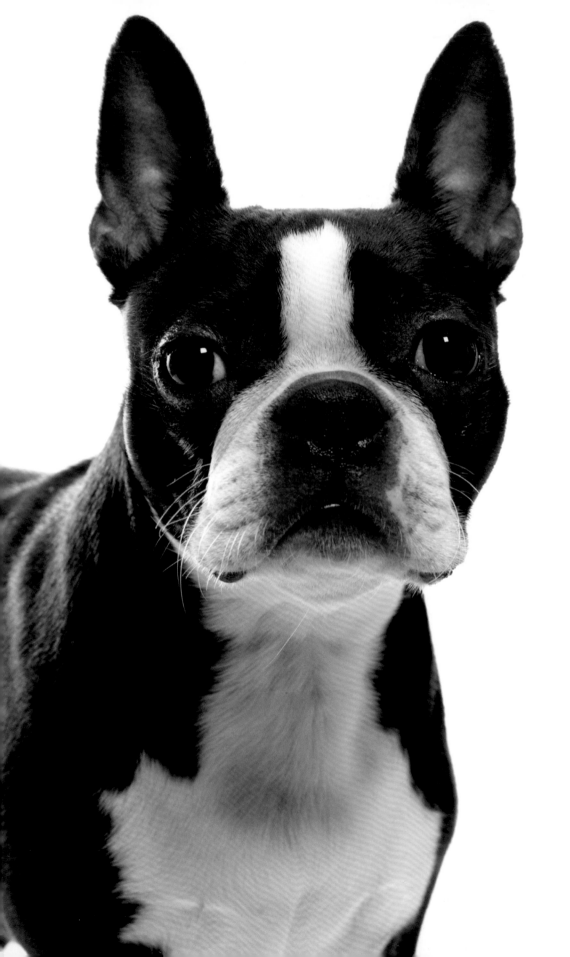

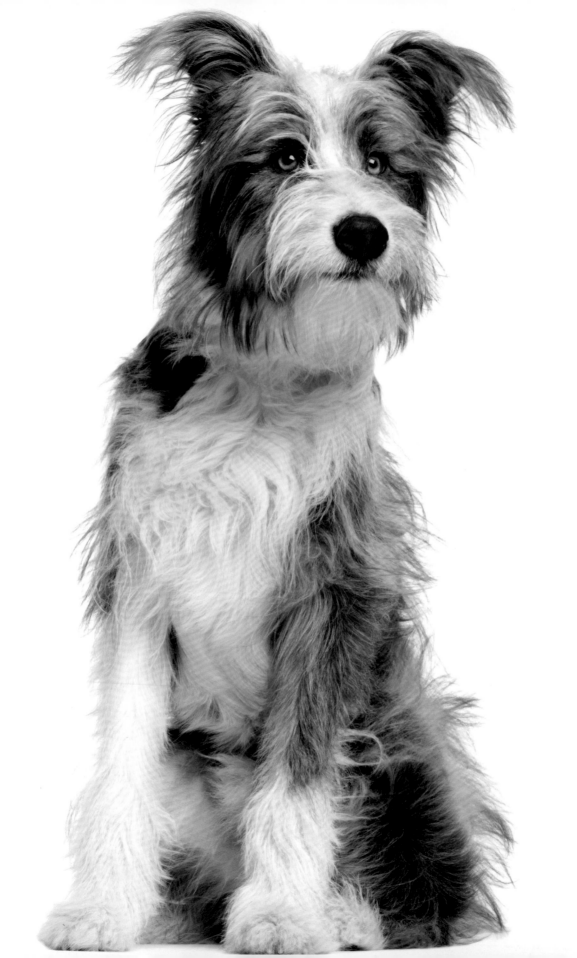

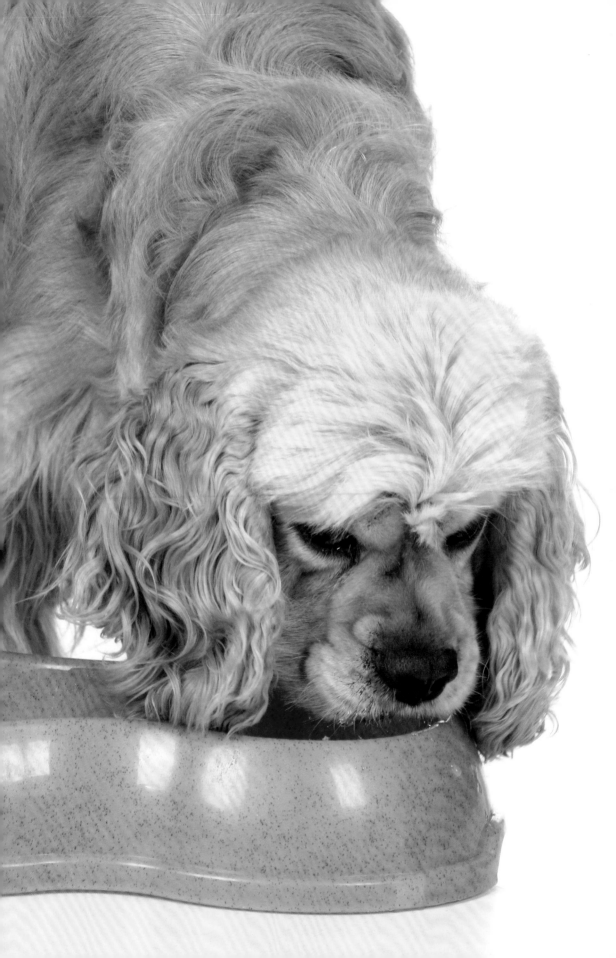

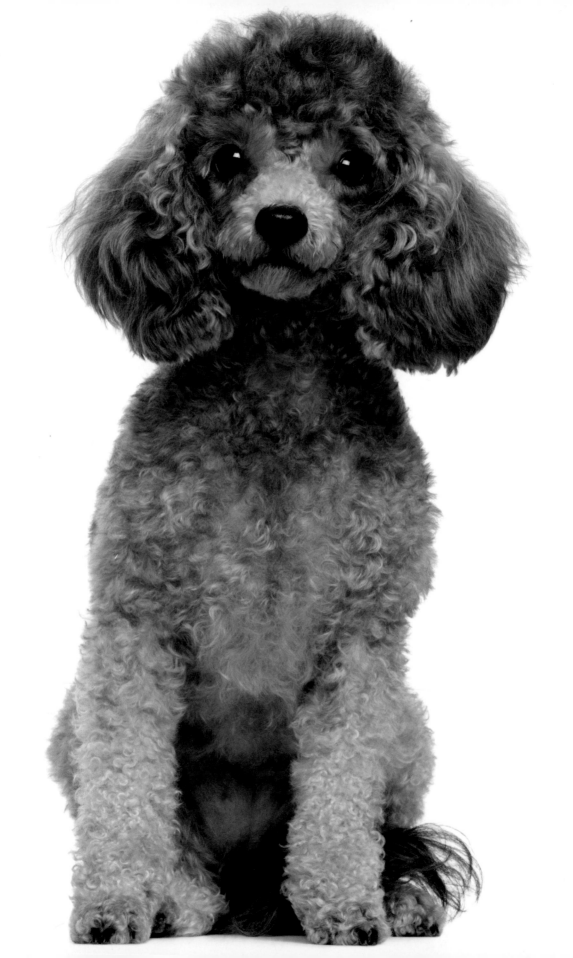

Tomato and Chicken Rotini

MAKES 1 SERVING

1 tbsp	canola oil	15 mL
1½ cups	cubed (½ inch/1 cm) boneless skinless chicken thighs	375 mL
⅔ cup	finely chopped tomato	150 mL
¼ cup	finely chopped zucchini	50 mL
¼ cup	tomato sauce	50 mL
2 tbsp	finely chopped green bell pepper	25 mL
½ tsp	dried basil leaves	2 mL
½ tsp	dried oregano leaves	2 mL
½ tsp	minced garlic	2 mL
2 cups	drained cooked rotini	500 mL
¼ tsp	potassium chloride (salt substitute)	1 mL
	Bonemeal and multivitamin-and-mineral supplements (see Chapter 7, page 206)	

1. In a saucepan, heat oil over medium heat. Add chicken and cook, stirring, until no longer pink inside. Stir in tomato, zucchini, tomato sauce, green pepper, basil, oregano and garlic. Cover and cook, stirring occasionally, for 10 minutes or until vegetables are soft.

2. Transfer to a serving bowl. Add rotini and mix thoroughly. Let cool until just warm to the touch. Stir in potassium chloride and supplements. Serve immediately.

• •

Nutritional Analysis *(Per Serving)*

1,154 kcal	98.8 g Carbohydrates
93.2 g Protein	36 g Fat

130 LBS | *58.9* KG

BASIC RECIPE •

Lamb and Rice

MAKES 4 SERVINGS	7¼ cups	cubed cooked lean boneless lamb	1.8 L
	6¾ cups	cooked long-grain brown rice	1.675 L
	6½ cups	pureed vegetable-and-fruit mix	1.625 L
	5 tbsp	canola oil	70 mL
	1 tsp	iodized salt	5 mL
	1 tsp	potassium chloride (salt substitute)	5 mL

This recipe should be divided into 4 servings, each containing approximately 1,177 kcal, or half the daily requirement. To meet your dog's nutritional needs, feed 2 servings a day.

Bonemeal and multivitamin-and-mineral supplements (see Chapter 7, page 206)

1. In a bowl, combine lamb, rice, vegetable-and-fruit mix, oil, salt and potassium chloride. Mix thoroughly. Divide into 4 equal portions.

2. Stir supplements into 1 portion and serve immediately. Cover and refrigerate or freeze the remaining portions. Stir supplements into each portion just before serving.

Tips

For basic instructions on how to cook the meats and carbohydrates, see pages 89 to 91.

For information on how to prepare the vegetable-and-fruit mix, see page 88.

For information on additional protein or carbohydrate substitutions, see page 87.

Cubes are ½ inch (1 cm).

The daily caloric requirement of a 130-lb (58.9 kg) dog ranges from 2,340 to 2,809 kcal.

• •

Nutritional Analysis *(Per Serving)*

1,177 kcal	**109 g Carbohydrates**
87.9 g Protein	**42.9 g Fat**

Variations

- **Beef and Rice:** Substitute 6¾ cups (1.675 L) drained cooked lean ground beef for the lamb.
- **Chicken and Rice:** Substitute 10 cups (2.5 L) cubed cooked boneless skinless chicken breast for the lamb.
- **Turkey and Rice:** Substitute 10½ cups (2.625 L) cubed cooked boneless skinless turkey breast for the lamb.
- **Meat and Macaroni:** Use the appropriate amount of your preferred meat and substitute 7½ cups (1.875 L) drained cooked macaroni for the rice.
- **Meat and Potatoes:** Use the appropriate amount of your preferred meat and substitute 12¼ cups (3.05 L) cubed peeled boiled potatoes for the rice. Omit potassium chloride.

GOURMET RECIPE •

Cottage Cheese, Fruit and Toast

MAKES 1 SERVING

Tip

If your dog consumes a milk product without previous exposure to dairy foods, low-level diarrhea may result. To properly break down and digest dairy products, your dog needs an enzyme called lactase, which must be developed gradually. To improve his/her ability to tolerate dairy products, add a small amount of yogurt or cottage cheese to any of the Basic Recipes. After a few weeks, your dog should be able to enjoy the calcium-rich foods from the dairy group and will lap up tasty breakfasts, such as Cottage Cheese, Fruit and Toast.

3	hard-boiled eggs, peeled and chopped	3
5½	slices whole wheat toast, torn into bite-size pieces	5½
1¼ cups	2% cottage cheese	300 mL
¾ cup	blueberries, thawed if frozen	175 mL
½ cup	diced cored apple	125 mL
¼ cup	chopped peeled banana	50 mL
1½ tbsp	canola oil	22 mL
¼ tsp	potassium chloride (salt substitute)	1 mL
	Bonemeal and multivitamin-and-mineral supplements (see Chapter 7, page 206)	

1. In a serving bowl, combine eggs, toast, cottage cheese, blueberries, apple, banana, oil, potassium chloride and supplements. Mix thoroughly. Serve immediately.

• •

Nutritional Analysis *(Per Serving)*

1,207 kcal	116.4 g Carbohydrates
74.8 g Protein	49.2 g Fat

Chow Time

Zoee's routine always involves food, and her feeding and cookie times are timed to the minute. As she weighs 90 pounds, Zoee can be quite persuasive when she wants something. She guides David and Jennifer to the fridge, the dinner bowls, the outside door or the cookie jar. Then she politely pushes them to Get to It! On those mornings when she pushes them toward the fridge, they know Zoee wants Cottage Cheese, Fruit and Toast for breakfast...NOW!

GOURMET RECIPE •

Red Snapper Stew

MAKES 1 SERVING			
	2 tbsp	canola oil	25 mL
	2¾ cups	cubed (½ inch/1 cm) boneless skinless red snapper	675 mL
	3 cups	cubed (½ inch/1 cm) peeled boiled potatoes	750 mL
	1½ cups	water	375 mL
	¾ cup	chopped green beans, thawed if frozen	175 mL
	½ cup	green peas, thawed if frozen	125 mL
	⅓ cup	finely chopped carrot	75 mL
	½ tsp	minced garlic	2 mL
	¼ tsp	iodized salt	1 mL
	¼ tsp	dried tarragon, thyme or basil leaves	1 mL
		Bonemeal and multivitamin-and-mineral supplements (see Chapter 7, page 206)	

1. In a saucepan, heat oil over medium-low heat. Add snapper and cook, stirring, until lightly browned. Add potatoes, water, green beans, peas, carrot, garlic, salt and tarragon. Cover and cook, stirring occasionally, for 10 minutes or until vegetables are soft. Let cool until just warm to the touch.

2. Stir in supplements. Transfer to a serving bowl. Serve immediately.

• •

Nutritional Analysis *(Per Serving)*

1,230 kcal	112.9 g Carbohydrates
121.4 g Protein	32.3 g Fat

GOURMET RECIPE •

Chicken Fricassee

MAKES 1 SERVING

1½ tbsp	canola oil	22 mL
2¼ cups	cubed (½ inch/1 cm) boneless skinless chicken breast	550 mL
⅓ cup	cubed (½ inch/1 cm) chicken livers	75 mL
½ tsp	minced garlic	2 mL
½ tsp	dried basil leaves	2 mL
½ tsp	dried oregano leaves	2 mL
¼ tsp	iodized salt	1 mL
2¾ cups	water	675 mL
3½ cups	cubed peeled potatoes	825 mL
¾ cup	finely chopped zucchini	175 mL
¾ cup	finely chopped tomato	175 mL
2 tbsp	finely chopped green bell pepper	25 mL
1 tsp	fresh lemon juice	5 mL
	Bonemeal and multivitamin-and-mineral supplements (see Chapter 7, page 206)	

1. In a nonstick skillet, heat oil over medium heat. Add chicken, chicken livers, garlic, basil, oregano and salt. Cook, stirring, until chicken is no longer pink inside. Add water and bring to a boil. Add potatoes. Reduce heat, cover and simmer for 15 minutes or until potatoes are tender.

2. Stir in zucchini, tomato, green pepper and lemon juice. Uncover and simmer, stirring occasionally, for 15 minutes or until vegetables are soft.

3. Let cool until just warm to the touch. Stir in supplements. Transfer to a serving bowl. Serve immediately.

• •

Nutritional Analysis *(Per Serving)*

1,241 kcal	119.6 g Carbohydrates
119.3 g Protein	30.8 g Fat

140 LBS | *63.4* KG

Beef and Rice

MAKES 4 SERVINGS			
7¼ cups	cooked long-grain brown rice		1.8 L
7 cups	drained cooked lean ground beef		1.75 L
7 cups	pureed vegetable-and-fruit mix		1.75 L
5½ tbsp	canola oil		75 mL
1 tsp	iodized salt		5 mL
1½ tsp	potassium chloride (salt substitute)		7 mL
	Bonemeal and multivitamin-and-mineral supplements (see Chapter 7, page 207)		

This recipe should be divided into 4 servings, each containing approximately 1,247 kcal, or half the daily requirement. To meet your dog's nutritional needs, feed 2 servings a day.

1. In a bowl, combine rice, beef, vegetable-and-fruit mix, oil, salt and potassium chloride. Mix thoroughly. Divide into 4 equal portions.

2. Stir supplements into 1 portion and serve immediately. Cover and refrigerate or freeze the remaining portions. Stir supplements into each portion just before serving.

Tips

For basic instructions on how to cook the meats and carbohydrates, see pages 89 to 91.

For information on how to prepare the vegetable-and-fruit mix, see page 88.

For information on additional protein or carbohydrate substitutions, see page 87.

Cubes are ½ inch (1 cm).

• •

Nutritional Analysis *(Per Serving)*

1,247 kcal	117.1 g Carbohydrates
67.1 g Protein	55.3 g Fat

Variations

- **Chicken and Rice:** Substitute 10½ cups (2.625 L) cubed cooked boneless skinless chicken breast for the beef.

- **Turkey and Rice:** Substitute 11 cups (2.75 L) cubed cooked boneless skinless turkey breast for the beef.

- **Lamb and Rice:** Substitute 7½ cups (1.875 L) cubed cooked lean boneless lamb for the beef.

- **Meat and Macaroni:** Use the appropriate amount of your preferred meat and substitute 8 cups (2 L) drained cooked macaroni for the rice.

- **Meat and Potatoes:** Use the appropriate amount of your preferred meat and substitute 13 cups (3.25 L) cubed peeled boiled potatoes for the rice. Omit potassium chloride.

> The daily caloric requirement of a 140-lb (63.4 kg) dog ranges from 2,474 to 2,969 kcal.

GOURMET RECIPE •

Oatmeal, Yogurt and Fruit

MAKES 1 SERVING

Tip

If your dog consumes a milk product without previous exposure to dairy foods, low-level diarrhea may result. To properly break down and digest dairy products, your dog needs an enzyme called lactase, which must be developed gradually. To improve his/her ability to tolerate dairy products, add a small amount of yogurt or cottage cheese to any of the Basic Recipes. After a few weeks, your dog should be able to enjoy the calcium-rich foods from the dairy group and will lap up tasty breakfasts, such as Oatmeal, Yogurt and Fruit.

3 cups	cooked rolled oats	750 mL
2¼ cups	non-fat yogurt	550 mL
1¼ cups	2% cottage cheese	300 mL
¾ cup	blueberries, thawed if frozen	175 mL
½ cup	diced cored apple	125 mL
⅓ cup	chopped peeled banana	75 mL
1½ tbsp	canola oil	22 mL
¼ tsp	potassium chloride (salt substitute)	1 mL
	Bonemeal and multivitamin-and-mineral supplements (see Chapter 7, page 207)	

1. In a serving bowl, combine oats, yogurt, cottage cheese, blueberries, apple, banana, oil, potassium chloride and supplements. Mix thoroughly. Serve immediately.

• •

Nutritional Analysis *(Per Serving)*

1,276 kcal	149.2 g Carbohydrates
90.4 g Protein	37.9 g Fat

Meals **167**

GOURMET RECIPE •

Barbecued Hamburgers

MAKES 1 SERVING

• *Preheat barbecue*

12 oz	lean ground beef	375 g
4	whole wheat hamburger buns	4
1 cup	finely chopped tomato	250 mL
1 cup	finely chopped lettuce	250 mL
1 tbsp	canola oil	15 mL
¼ tsp	potassium chloride (salt substitute)	1 mL
	Bonemeal and multivitamin-and-mineral supplements (see Chapter 7, page 207)	

1. Form beef into four ½-inch (1 cm) thick patties. Place on preheated barbecue and grill, turning once, until no longer pink inside. Let cool until just warm to the touch.

2. Cut burgers and buns into bite-size pieces. In a serving bowl, combine burgers, buns, tomato, lettuce, oil, potassium chloride and supplements. Mix thoroughly. Serve immediately.

• •

Nutritional Analysis *(Per Serving)*

1,414 kcal	116.3 g Carbohydrates
96.1 g Protein	63 g Fat

GOURMET RECIPE •

Salmon and Dill Pasta

MAKES 1 SERVING			
1½ tbsp	canola oil	22 mL
12 oz	cubed (½ inch/1 cm) boneless skinless salmon	375 g
¾ cup	finely chopped tomato	175 mL
¾ cup	finely chopped zucchini	175 mL
½ cup	finely chopped spinach	125 mL
½ tsp	minced garlic	2 mL
¼ tsp	dried dillweed	1 mL
¼ tsp	iodized salt	1 mL
2¼ cups	drained cooked rotini or macaroni	550 mL
	Bonemeal and multivitamin-and-mineral supplements (see Chapter 7, page 207)	

1. In a saucepan, heat oil over medium-low heat. Add salmon and cook, stirring, until fish flakes easily when tested with a fork. Reduce heat to low and add tomato, zucchini, spinach, garlic, dill and salt. Cook, stirring, for 5 minutes or until vegetables are soft. Transfer to a serving bowl. Add rotini and mix thoroughly. Let cool until just warm to the touch.

2. Stir in supplements. Serve immediately.

• •

Nutritional Analysis *(Per Serving)*

1,247 kcal	107.7 g Carbohydrates
92.7 g Protein	48.5 g Fat

Please Eat the Salmon

Shortly after David and Jennifer adopted Dylan, they were having salmon for lunch. When they offered him a piece, he gently took it in his mouth, dropped it on the floor and promptly rolled on it. Since then, Dylan has come to appreciate that eating salmon is more enjoyable than rolling on it. However, they still need to keep a close eye on him while walking on the beach.

150 LBS | *68.0* KG

BASIC RECIPE •

Chicken and Rice

MAKES 4 SERVINGS

This recipe should be divided into 4 servings, each containing approximately 1,320 kcal, or half the daily requirement. To meet your dog's nutritional needs, feed 2 servings a day.

11¼ cups	cubed cooked boneless skinless chicken breast	2.8 L
7½ cups	cooked long-grain brown rice	1.875 L
7¼ cups	pureed vegetable-and-fruit mix	1.8 L
⅓ cup	canola oil	75 mL
1 tsp	iodized salt	5 mL
1½ tsp	potassium chloride (salt substitute)	7 mL
	Bonemeal and multivitamin-and-mineral supplements (see Chapter 7, page 207)	

Tips

For basic instructions on how to cook the meats and carbohydrates, see pages 89 to 91.

For information on how to prepare the vegetable-and-fruit mix, see page 88.

For information on additional protein or carbohydrate substitutions, see page 87.

Cubes are ½ inch (1 cm).

1. In a bowl, combine chicken, rice, vegetable-and-fruit mix, oil, salt and potassium chloride. Mix thoroughly. Divide into 4 equal portions.

2. Stir supplements into 1 portion and serve immediately. Cover and refrigerate or freeze the remaining portions. Stir supplements into each portion just before serving.

• •

Nutritional Analysis *(Per Serving)*

1,320 kcal	**121.2 g Carbohydrates**
127.7 g Protein	**33.4 g Fat**

The daily caloric requirement of a 150-lb (68.0 kg) dog ranges from 2,606 to 3,127 kcal.

Variations

- **Beef and Rice:** Substitute 7½ cups (1.875 L) drained cooked lean ground beef for the chicken.
- **Turkey and Rice:** Substitute 11¾ cups (2.925 L) cubed cooked boneless skinless turkey breast for the chicken.
- **Lamb and Rice:** Substitute 8 cups (2 L) cubed cooked lean boneless lamb for the chicken.
- **Meat and Macaroni:** Use the appropriate amount of your preferred meat and substitute 8½ cups (2.125 L) drained cooked macaroni for the rice.
- **Meat and Potatoes:** Use the appropriate amount of your preferred meat and substitute 13½ cups (3.375 L) cubed peeled boiled potatoes for the rice. Omit potassium chloride.

GOURMET RECIPE •

Steak, Eggs and Hash Browns

MAKES 1 SERVING

12 oz	cubed (½ inch/1 cm) top sirloin steak	375 g
1½ tbsp	canola oil	22 mL
3	large eggs, beaten	3
¾ cup	finely chopped tomato	175 mL
¾ cup	chopped green beans, thawed if frozen	175 mL
2 tbsp	finely chopped green bell pepper	25 mL
½ tsp	minced garlic	2 mL
½ tsp	dried basil leaves	2 mL
¼ tsp	iodized salt	1 mL
3½ cups	cubed (½ inch/1 cm) peeled boiled potatoes	825 mL
	Bonemeal and multivitamin-and-mineral supplements (see Chapter 7, page 207)	

1. In a nonstick skillet, cook steak over medium heat until no longer pink inside. Transfer to a serving bowl. Let cool. Wipe skillet clean.

2. In same skillet, heat oil over medium heat. Add eggs, tomato, green beans, green pepper, garlic, basil and salt. Cook, stirring, for 8 minutes or until vegetables are soft and eggs are just set. Let cool until just warm to the touch.

3. Add egg mixture, potatoes and supplements to steak. Mix thoroughly. Serve immediately.

• •

Nutritional Analysis *(Per Serving)*

1,418 kcal	126.3 g Carbohydrates
104.3 g Protein	54.4 g Fat

GOURMET RECIPE •

Basil Chicken and Vegetable Pasta

MAKES 1 SERVING		
1½ tbsp	canola oil	22 mL
2¾ cups	cubed (½ inch/1 cm) boneless skinless chicken breast	675 mL
½ tsp	minced garlic	2 mL
¾ cup	finely chopped tomato	175 mL
¾ cup	finely chopped zucchini	175 mL
2 tbsp	finely chopped green bell pepper	25 mL
2½ cups	drained cooked rotini or macaroni	625 mL
1½ tbsp	finely chopped fresh basil leaves (or 1½ tsp/7 mL dried basil leaves)	22 mL
¼ tsp	potassium chloride (salt substitute)	1 mL
¼ tsp	iodized salt	1 mL
1 tsp	freshly grated Parmesan cheese (optional)	5 mL
	Bonemeal and multivitamin-and-mineral supplements (see Chapter 7, page 207)	

1. In a large nonstick skillet, heat oil over medium heat. Add chicken and garlic. Cook, stirring, until chicken is no longer pink inside. Add tomato, zucchini and green pepper. Cook, stirring, for 6 minutes or until vegetables are soft.

2. Remove from heat and stir in rotini, basil, potassium chloride and salt. Stir in Parmesan cheese, if using. Let cool until just warm to the touch.

3. Stir in supplements. Transfer to a serving bowl. Serve immediately.

• •

Nutritional Analysis *(Per Serving)*

1,324 kcal	118.8 g Carbohydrates
133.3 g Protein	31.5 g Fat

GOURMET RECIPE •

Stir-Fried Ginger Beef
with Greens

MAKES 1 SERVING

• Wok

2 tbsp	canola oil	25 mL
1 lb	top sirloin steak, cut into ½-inch (1 cm) cubes	500 g
1 tsp	minced gingerroot	5 mL
½ tsp	minced garlic	2 mL
¾ cup	chopped green beans, thawed if frozen	175 mL
½ cup	green peas, thawed if frozen	125 mL
½ cup	finely chopped spinach	125 mL
1½ tbsp	light soy sauce	22 mL
2 cups	cooked long-grain brown rice	500 mL
¼ tsp	potassium chloride (salt substitute)	1 mL
	Bonemeal and multivitamin-and-mineral supplements (see Chapter 7, page 207)	

1. In a wok or nonstick skillet, heat oil over medium heat. Add steak, ginger and garlic. Cook, stirring, until steak is no longer pink inside. Add green beans, peas, spinach and soy sauce. Cook, stirring frequently, for 4 minutes or until vegetables are soft. Transfer to a serving bowl.

2. Add rice. Let cool until just warm to the touch. Stir potassium chloride and supplements. Serve immediately.

• •

Nutritional Analysis *(Per Serving)*

1,395 kcal	113.9 g Carbohydrates
106.7 g Protein	55.9 g Fat

The Global Diner
If your dog is a culinary adventurer, try this flavorful adaptation of a classic Chinese dish.

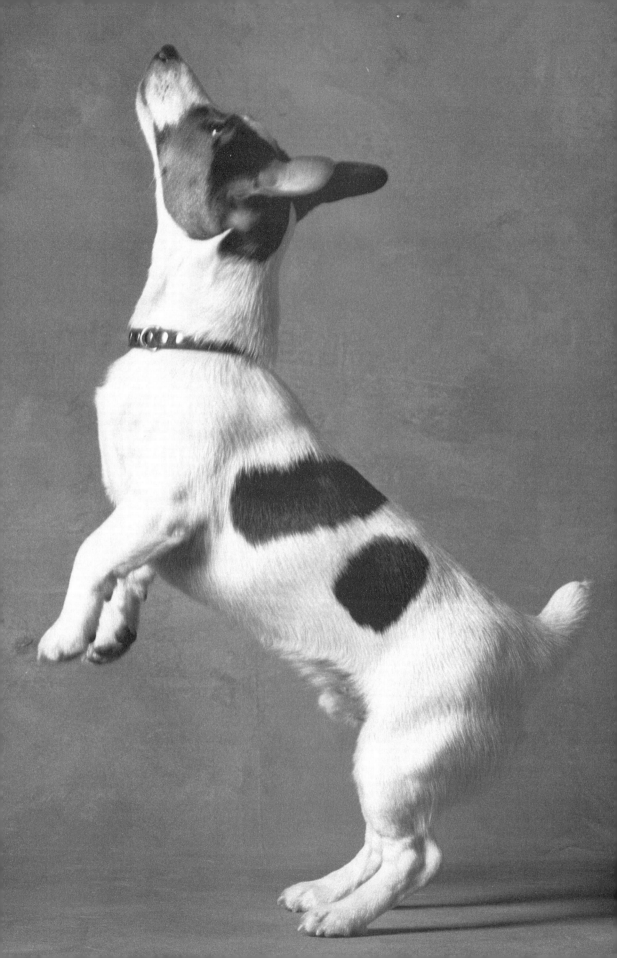

CHAPTER SIX

Cookies

Max's Veggie Cookies

**MAKES ABOUT
1 LB (500 G) OF COOKIES**

Tip

Over the years, one of the lessons we've learned is that dogs don't care about the shape of their cookies. They're only interested in the taste. We recommend cutting cookies into squares because it's easy. But if you have cookie cutters, feel free to use them — with one word of caution: take care to ensure that the size and shape of the cookie is safe for the size of your dog. For instance, if the cookies are small and round, your dog may not chew them enough — and may even swallow them whole, which could lead to choking. Since cookies are hard, shapes with sharp pointy edges, such as stars, may cut your dog's mouth or become lodged in his/her esophagus.

- Preheat oven to 350°F (180°C)
- Nonstick baking sheets • Food processor
- Rolling pin • Pizza cutter

4 cups	whole wheat flour	1 L
1 tsp	dried basil leaves	5 mL
1 tsp	dried cilantro leaves	5 mL
1 tsp	dried oregano leaves	5 mL
¾ cup	water	175 mL
⅔ cup	chopped carrot	150 mL
¼ cup	cut (½ inch/1 cm) green beans, thawed if frozen	50 mL
2 tbsp	each tomato paste	25 mL
2 tbsp	canola oil	25 mL
1	clove garlic	1

1. In a large bowl, combine flour, basil, cilantro and oregano. In a food processor, combine water, carrot, green beans, tomato paste, oil and garlic. Puree until smooth. Pour over dry ingredients and mix well.

2. In the bowl and using hands, knead until dough holds together. Transfer to lightly floured surface. Using a rolling pin, roll out dough to about ⅛-inch (3 mm) thickness.

3. With a fork, poke holes all over the surface of the dough. Using a pizza cutter or a sharp knife, cut dough into bite-size rectangles or squares. Place about ½ inch (1 cm) apart on baking sheets.

4. Bake in preheated oven, in batches if necessary, for 20 minutes or until firm. Place pans on racks and let cool completely. Reduce oven temperature to 300°F (150°C). Bake for 30 minutes longer or until hard. Transfer cookies to a rack and let cool completely. Store in a tightly sealed container for up to 30 days.

Variation

- **Low-Fat Veggie Cookies:** For a lower-fat version of this cookie recipe, replace the canola oil with 2 tbsp (25 mL) of additional water.

A Tribute to Max

Years ago, just before a thunderstorm broke, an old, lumbering Lab named Max appeared at the front door of the bakery. He was panting and in a state of high anxiety, so David and Jennifer invited him to stay until the storm was over. Subsequently, Max decided that the bakery was a refuge and, for the next six years, he was a regular. He visited when his family was at work or during storms and forest fires. Often, he came just to hang out. His charming antics made many people smile, and everyone enjoyed having him around. This was his favorite cookie. He is greatly missed.

Dylan's Blueberry Peach and Flax Cookies

**MAKES ABOUT
1 LB (500 G) OF COOKIES**

- Preheat oven to 350°F (180°C)
- Nonstick baking sheets • Food processor
- Rolling pin • Pizza cutter

4 cups	whole wheat flour	1 L
2 tbsp	flaxseeds	25 mL
½ tsp	ground cinnamon	2 mL
1 cup	water	250 mL
⅓ cup	blueberries, thawed if frozen	75 mL
3 tbsp	finely chopped peeled peaches, thawed if frozen	45 mL
2 tbsp	liquid honey	25 mL
2 tbsp	canola oil	25 mL
1	large egg	1
1 tsp	vanilla	5 mL

1. In a large bowl, combine flour, flaxseeds and cinnamon. In a food processor, combine water, blueberries, peaches, honey, oil, egg and vanilla. Puree until smooth. Pour over dry ingredients and stir until well incorporated.

2. In the bowl and using hands, knead until dough holds together. Transfer to lightly floured surface. Using a rolling pin, roll out dough to about ⅛-inch (3 mm) thickness.

3. With a fork, poke holes all over the surface of the dough. Using a pizza cutter or a sharp knife, cut dough into bite-size rectangles or squares. Place about ½ inch (1 cm) apart on baking sheets.

4. Bake in preheated oven, in batches if necessary, for 20 minutes or until firm. Place pans on racks and let cool completely. Reduce oven temperature to 300°F (150°C). Bake for 30 minutes longer or until hard. Transfer cookies to a rack and let cool completely. Store in a tightly sealed container for up to 30 days.

The Lifesaver

David and Jennifer are certain that the smell of these delicious cookies saved Dylan's life. They often saw him walking past the bakery when he wandered away from his former home, but they couldn't get near him because he was fearful of people. One day, when a batch of these cookies was baking, Dylan came as far as the front door, sniffing. When they got too close, he ran off, but the incident motivated them to leave cookies and water out for him on a regular basis. One day, on a visit to the animal shelter, Jennifer recognized Dylan, who had been picked up for running at large. His former significant humans no longer wanted him — they had a new puppy — and Dylan was about to be destroyed. Thanks to these cookies, which brought him to the bakery, Jennifer recognized Dylan at the shelter and she and David made him a welcome part of their family.

Mom's Famous Pumpkin Biscotti

**MAKES ABOUT
1 LB (500 G) OF BISCOTTI**

- *Preheat oven to 350°F (180°C)*
- *Nonstick baking sheets*

1 cup	canned pumpkin puree (not pie filling)	250 mL
1/4 cup	each liquid honey and water	50 mL
2 tbsp	canola oil	25 mL
1	large egg	1
1 tsp	vanilla	5 mL
4 cups	all-purpose flour	1 L
1 tsp	ground cinnamon	5 mL
1/4 tsp	baking powder	1 mL
1/4 tsp	baking soda	1 mL

1. In a large bowl, whisk together pumpkin puree, honey, water, oil, egg and vanilla. Stir in flour, cinnamon, baking powder and baking soda until well incorporated.

2. In the bowl and using hands, knead until dough holds together. Transfer to lightly floured surface. Divide dough into 2 equal pieces. Shape each piece into a log. Flatten the logs to make about 4 inches (10 cm) wide.

3. With a fork, poke holes all over the surface of the logs. Place about 4 inches (10 cm) apart on baking sheet.

4. Bake in preheated oven for 35 to 40 minutes or until firm. Place pan on a rack and let cool for 30 minutes. Reduce oven temperature to 300°F (150°C).

5. With a sharp knife, cut each log into ¼-inch (0.5 cm) thick slices. Place, cut side down, about ½ inch (1 cm) apart on baking sheets. Bake for 30 minutes longer or until hard. Transfer cookies to a rack and let cool completely. Store in a tightly sealed container for up to 30 days.

I Can Believe I Ate the Whole Thing

One Thanksgiving, Grant's parents arrived for dinner with a plate of his mom's famous Pumpkin Biscotti. When dessert time arrived, no one could find the biscotti, and dinner was concluded without the tasty treat. Grant didn't find the empty plate until the next morning. It was in the backyard, complete with a licked-clean doily. Otis was looking particularly pleased with himself, as well he might since it was a job well done. Somehow, he managed to transport the entire plate of biscotti down a flight of stairs, through the dog door and into the yard, where he ate the whole thing.

Carrot Apple Oatmeal Flax Cookies

- *Preheat oven to 350°F (180°C)*
- *Nonstick baking sheets • Food processor*
- *Rolling pin • Pizza cutter*

3 cups	whole wheat flour	750 mL
1 cup	quick-cooking rolled oats	250 mL
2 tbsp	flaxseeds	25 mL
½ tsp	ground cinnamon	2 mL
¾ cup	water	175 mL
½ cup	chopped carrot	125 mL
¼ cup	finely chopped cored apple	50 mL
2 tbsp	each blackstrap molasses and canola oil	25 mL
1	large egg	1
1 tsp	vanilla	5 mL

1. In a large bowl, combine flour, oats, flaxseeds and cinnamon. In a food processor, combine water, carrot, apple, molasses, oil, egg and vanilla. Puree until smooth. Pour over dry ingredients and mix well.

2. In the bowl and using hands, knead until dough holds together. Transfer to lightly floured surface. Using a rolling pin, roll out dough to about ⅛-inch (3 mm) thickness. With a fork, poke holes all over the surface of the dough. Using a pizza cutter or a sharp knife, cut dough into bite-size rectangles or squares. Place about ½ inch (1 cm) apart on baking sheets.

3. Bake in preheated oven, in batches if necessary, for 20 minutes or until firm. Place pans on racks and let cool completely. Reduce oven temperature to 300°F (150°C). Bake for 30 minutes longer or until hard. Transfer cookies to a rack and let cool completely. Store in a tightly sealed container for up to 30 days.

> **Try This**
> This is one of the most popular cookies at Licks and Wags Bakery.

Barley Banana Cookies

Tip
These delicious cookies have a hard, crunchy texture that provides abrasion for the teeth, which benefits your dog's oral health.

- *Preheat oven to 350°F (180°C)*
- *Nonstick baking sheets • Food processor*
- *Rolling pin • Pizza cutter*

2 cups	whole wheat flour	500 mL
2 cups	barley flour	500 mL
½ cup	brown rice flour	125 mL
1 cup	chopped peeled banana	250 mL
½ cup	water	125 mL
2 tbsp	canola oil	25 mL
1	large egg	1
2 tsp	blackstrap molasses	10 mL

1. In a large bowl, combine whole wheat, barley and brown rice flours. In a food processor, combine banana, water, oil, egg and molasses. Puree until smooth. Pour over dry ingredients and stir until well incorporated.

2. In the bowl and using hands, knead until dough holds together. Transfer to lightly floured surface. Using a rolling pin, roll out dough to about ⅛-inch (3 mm) thickness.

3. With a fork, poke holes all over the surface of the dough. Using a pizza cutter or a sharp knife, cut dough into bite-size rectangles or squares. Place about ½ inch (1 cm) apart on baking sheets.

4. Bake in preheated oven, in batches if necessary, for 18 minutes or until firm. Place pans on racks and let cool completely. Reduce oven temperature to 300°F (150°C). Bake for 30 minutes longer or until hard. Transfer cookies to a rack and let cool completely. Store in a tightly sealed container for up to 30 days.

A Universal Favorite
Here's a great flavor combination that all our dogs enjoy.

Peanut Butter Cookies

**MAKES ABOUT
1 LB (500 G) OF COOKIES**

Tip
Poking holes in the dough (which is called docking) ensures that the cookies won't get puffy. If you have a genuine docking wheel, by all means use it. But a fork works well, too.

- Preheat oven to 350°F (180°C)
- Nonstick baking sheets
- Rolling pin • Pizza cutter

1 cup + 1 tbsp	water	265 mL
1 cup	smooth natural peanut butter	250 mL
1	large egg	1
1 tsp	vanilla	5 mL
4 cups	whole wheat flour	1 L
½ cup	cornmeal	125 mL

1. In a large bowl, whisk together water, peanut butter, egg and vanilla. Stir in flour and cornmeal until well incorporated.

2. In the bowl and using hands, knead until dough holds together. Transfer to lightly floured surface. Using a rolling pin, roll out dough to about ⅛-inch (3 mm) thickness.

3. With a fork, poke holes all over the surface of the dough. Using a pizza cutter or a sharp knife, cut dough into bite-size rectangles or squares. Place about ½ inch (1 cm) apart on baking sheets.

4. Bake in preheated oven, in batches if necessary, for 18 minutes or until firm. Place pans on racks and let cool completely. Reduce oven temperature to 300°F (150°C). Bake for 20 minutes longer or until hard. Transfer cookies to a rack and let cool completely. Store in a tightly sealed container for up to 30 days.

Not Just on Toast
Before David and Jennifer started baking their own cookies, their dog Harris turned his nose up at most treats. They were pretty sure he would like these, as he loves peanut butter on toast. They were right.

Barley Apple Cinnamon Cookies

**MAKES ABOUT
1 LB (500 G) OF COOKIES**

- *Preheat oven to 350°F (180°C)*
- *Nonstick baking sheets • Food processor*
- *Rolling pin • Pizza cutter*

2 cups	barley flour	500 mL
2 cups	whole wheat flour	500 mL
1 tsp	ground cinnamon	5 mL
1 cup	water	250 mL
½ cup	chopped cored apple	125 mL
2 tbsp	canola oil	25 mL
2 tbsp	blackstrap molasses	25 mL
1	large egg	1

1. In a large bowl, combine barley and whole wheat flours and cinnamon. In a food processor, combine water, apple, oil, molasses and egg. Puree until smooth. Pour over dry ingredients and stir until well incorporated.

2. In the bowl and using hands, knead until dough holds together. Transfer to lightly floured surface. Using a rolling pin, roll out dough to about ⅛-inch (3 mm) thickness.

3. With a fork, poke holes all over the surface of the dough. Using a pizza cutter or a sharp knife, cut dough into bite-size rectangles or squares. Place about ½ inch (1 cm) apart on baking sheets.

4. Bake in preheated oven, in batches if necessary, for 20 minutes or until firm. Place pans on racks and let cool completely. Reduce oven temperature to 300°F (150°C). Bake for 30 minutes longer or until hard. Transfer cookies to a rack and let cool completely. Store in a tightly sealed container for up to 30 days.

Just Like Mom's Apple Pie
Apples and cinnamon are an unbeatable combination. You'll love the smell that wafts through the house while these cookies bake, and your dog will love their delicious taste.

Carrot and Cinnamon Cookies

**MAKES ABOUT
1 LB (500 G) OF COOKIES**

- *Preheat oven to 350°F (180°C)*
- *Nonstick baking sheets • Food processor*
- *Rolling pin • Pizza cutter*

4 cups	whole wheat flour	1 L
½ cup	cornmeal	125 mL
1 tsp	ground cinnamon	5 mL
1 cup	chopped carrot	250 mL
½ cup	water	125 mL
2 tbsp	canola oil	25 mL
2 tbsp	liquid honey	25 mL
1	large egg	1
1 tsp	vanilla	5 mL

1. In a large bowl, combine flour, cornmeal and cinnamon. In a food processor, combine carrot, water, oil, honey, egg and vanilla. Puree until smooth. Pour over dry ingredients and stir until well incorporated.

2. In the bowl and using hands, knead until dough holds together. Transfer to lightly floured surface. Using a rolling pin, roll out dough to about ⅛-inch (3 mm) thickness.

3. With a fork, poke holes all over the surface of the dough. Using a pizza cutter or a sharp knife, cut dough into bite-size rectangles or squares. Place about ½ inch (1 cm) apart on baking sheets.

4. Bake in preheated oven, in batches if necessary, for 20 minutes or until firm. Place pans on racks and let cool completely. Reduce oven temperature to 300°F (150°C). Bake for 30 minutes longer or until hard. Transfer cookies to a rack and let cool completely. Store in a tightly sealed container for up to 30 days.

Variation

● **Low-Fat Carrot and Cinnamon Cookies:** For a lower-fat version of this cookie recipe, replace the canola oil with 2 tbsp (25 mL) of additional water.

A Happy Ending

At Licks and Wags, David and Jennifer often receive mail from satisfied customers. One letter came from a couple who adopted an emaciated dog they found on the side of a highway. They tried everything to get her to eat, with no success. Then a friend brought them a bag of Licks and Wags Carrot and Cinnamon Cookies. The dog loved the cookies, so they started adding broken bits of them to her food. At first she extracted the cookie bits, but gradually she began to eat the food as well and eventually was consuming a normal amount. Her significant humans thanked David and Jennifer for baking the cookies that saved their new dog's life, and that made them feel very good.

Oatmeal Peach Cookies

MAKES ABOUT 1½ LBS (750 G) OF COOKIES

• Preheat oven to 350°F (180°C)
• Nonstick baking sheets • Food processor
• Rolling pin • Pizza cutter

Tip

This dough is very soft and easy to roll out. We recommend rolling the dough this thinly because the edges will burn and the middles will be soft if it is too thick.

4 cups	quick-cooking rolled oats	1 L
1½ cups	water, divided	375 mL
½ cup	finely chopped peeled peaches, thawed if frozen	125 mL
2 tbsp	canola oil	25 mL
2 tbsp	blackstrap molasses	25 mL
½ tsp	vanilla	2 mL
2 cups	whole wheat flour	500 mL
1 tsp	ground cinnamon	5 mL

1. In a large bowl, soak oats in 1⅛ cups (275 mL) water for 10 minutes.

2. Meanwhile, in a food processor, combine peaches, ¼ cup (50 mL) water, oil, molasses and vanilla. Puree until smooth. Stir into oat mixture along with remaining water, flour and cinnamon until well incorporated.

3. In the bowl and using hands, knead until dough holds together. Transfer to lightly floured surface. Using a rolling pin, roll out dough to about 1/16-inch (2 mm) thickness.

4. With a fork, poke holes all over the surface of the dough. Using a pizza cutter or a sharp knife, cut dough into bite-size rectangles or squares. Place about ½ inch (1 cm) apart on baking sheets.

5. Bake in preheated oven, in batches if necessary, for 16 minutes or until firm. Place pans on racks and let cool completely. Reduce oven temperature to 300°F (150°C). Bake for 20 minutes longer or until hard. Transfer cookies to a rack and let cool completely. Store in a tightly sealed container for up to 30 days.

Blueberry Banana Biscotti

**MAKES ABOUT
1 LB (500 G) OF BISCOTTI**

- Preheat oven to 350°F (180°C)
- Nonstick baking sheets • Food processor

4 cups	all-purpose flour	1 L
¼ tsp	baking powder	1 mL
¼ tsp	baking soda	1 mL
1 cup	chopped peeled banana	250 mL
½ cup	blueberries, thawed if frozen	125 mL
2 tbsp	each canola oil and water	25 mL
1	large egg	1
1 tsp	vanilla	5 mL

1. In a large bowl, combine flour, baking powder and baking soda. In a food processor, combine banana, blueberries, oil, water, egg and vanilla. Puree until smooth. Pour over dry ingredients and mix well.

2. In the bowl and using hands, knead until dough holds together. Transfer to lightly floured surface. Divide dough into 2 equal pieces. Shape each piece into a log. Flatten the logs to make about 4 inches (10 cm) wide.

3. With a fork, poke holes all over the surface of the logs. Place about 4 inches (10 cm) apart on baking sheet.

4. Bake in preheated oven for 35 to 40 minutes or until firm. Place pan on a rack and let cool for 30 minutes. Reduce oven temperature to 300°F (150°C).

5. With a sharp knife, cut each log into ¼-inch/0.5 cm thick slices. Place, cut side down, about ½ inch (1 cm) apart on baking sheets. Bake for 30 minutes longer or until hard. Transfer cookies to a rack and let cool completely. Store in a tightly sealed container for up to 30 days.

Zeus and the Italian Cookie
What would our beloved friend Zeus do without his biscotti? No one knows...and that's why we keep baking them for him! This is his favorite flavor.

Veggie Puppy Treats

**MAKES ABOUT
1 LB (500 G) OF TREATS**

- *Preheat oven to 350°F (180°C)*
- *Nonstick baking sheets • Food processor*
- *Rolling pin • Pizza cutter*

4 cups	whole wheat flour	1 L
1 tsp	each dried basil, cilantro and oregano leaves	5 mL
¾ cup	water	175 mL
⅔ cup	chopped carrot	150 mL
¼ cup	cut (½ inch/1 cm) green beans, thawed if frozen	50 mL
2 tbsp	tomato paste	25 mL
2 tbsp	canola oil	25 mL
1	clove garlic	1

1. In a large bowl, combine flour, basil, cilantro and oregano. In a food processor, combine water, carrot, green beans, tomato paste, oil and garlic. Puree until smooth. Pour over dry ingredients and mix well.

2. In the bowl and using hands, knead until dough holds together. Transfer to lightly floured surface. Using a rolling pin, roll out dough to about ⅛-inch (3 mm) thickness.

3. With a fork, poke holes all over the surface of the dough. Using a pizza cutter or a sharp knife, cut dough into ½-inch (1 cm) squares. Place about ½ inch (1 cm) apart on baking sheets.

4. Bake in preheated oven, in batches if necessary, for 20 minutes or until firm. Place pans on racks and let cool completely. Reduce oven temperature to 300°F (150°C). Bake for 25 minutes longer or until hard. Transfer cookies to a rack and let cool completely. Store in a tightly sealed container for up to 30 days.

Positive Reinforcement
Rewarding your puppy for good behavior with one of these delicious cookies will help him/her develop into a well-behaved dog.

Carrot and Cinnamon Puppy Treats

MAKES ABOUT 1 LB (500 G) OF TREATS

- Preheat oven to 350°F (180°C)
- Nonstick baking sheets • Food processor
- Rolling pin • Pizza cutter

4 cups	whole wheat flour	1 L
½ cup	cornmeal	125 mL
1 tsp	ground cinnamon	5 mL
1 cup	chopped carrot	250 mL
½ cup	water	125 mL
2 tbsp	each canola oil and liquid honey	25 mL
1	large egg	1
1 tsp	vanilla	5 mL

1. In a large bowl, combine flour, cornmeal and cinnamon. In a food processor, combine carrot, water, oil, honey, egg and vanilla. Puree until smooth. Pour over dry ingredients and stir until well incorporated.

2. In the bowl and using hands, knead until dough holds together. Transfer to lightly floured surface. Using a rolling pin, roll out dough to about ⅛-inch (3 mm) thickness. With a fork, poke holes all over the surface of the dough. Using a pizza cutter or a sharp knife, cut dough into ½-inch (1 cm) squares. Place about ½ inch (1 cm) apart on baking sheets.

3. Bake in preheated oven, in batches if necessary, for 20 minutes or until firm. Place pans on racks and let cool completely. Reduce oven temperature to 300°F (150°C). Bake for 25 minutes longer or until hard. Transfer cookies to a rack and let cool completely. Store in a tightly sealed container for up to 30 days.

Don't Wait Until All Else Fails

A dog trainer once said, "I don't care why your dog comes when you call, just that he does." We soon discovered that dogs respond well to bribery. Hence our popular If All Else Fails...Bribe M Bits™.

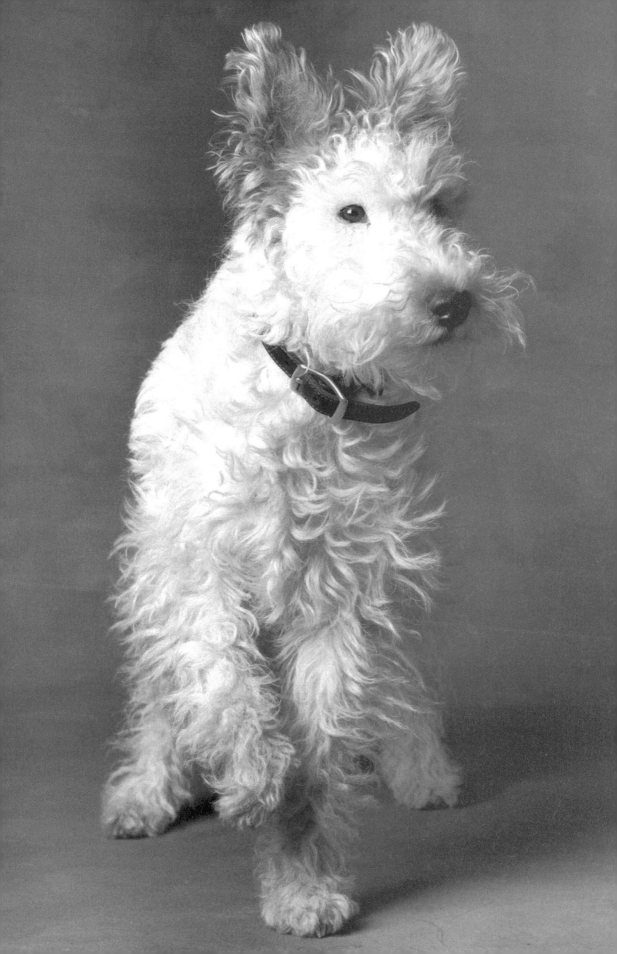

Adding Essential Nutrients

BENTLEY — 15-MONTH-OLD FOX TERRIER

The Supplements

IN THEORY, MOST OF YOUR DOG'S NUTRITIONAL NEEDS should be met by the recipes we have provided. However, some essential nutrients will be missing. Moreover, as it is virtually impossible to precisely define the nutrient value of foods given the unreliability of the food supply, as noted earlier, supplements are needed to ensure that your dog's nutritional needs are met. To properly supplement your dog's diet, you will need to purchase both bonemeal and a multivitamin-and-mineral supplement. These additional nutrients should be added daily according to the chart that corresponds to your dog's weight class.

Using the Charts

When using these charts, keep in mind that the levels noted are daily minimum requirements, which means that it is essential that your dog's diet provide at least this level of nutrients. While it may seem that the diet provides most of the nutrients your dog needs, supplementation is still necessary. Otherwise, nutritional deficiencies will result.

The sample recipe that the charts are based on is Beef and Rice, which contains lean ground beef, brown rice, vegetable-and-fruit mix, canola oil, iodized salt and potassium chloride (salt substitute). This recipe is fairly typical of the recipes in the book, except that it makes two servings. Although there will be variations in nutrient levels depending on the ingredients used, the addition of bonemeal and a good multivitamin-and-mineral supplement suitable for use with a home-prepared diet, ensures that any variations among the recipes are addressed.

> ## *Half per Meal*
>
> The charts are based on a dog's nutritional requirements for a full day, so it is important to supplement only half of the recommended amounts, twice a day, at each meal.

Bonemeal

Bonemeal provides calcium and phosphorus, which should be present in a ratio of approximately 2 parts calcium to 1 part phosphorus. Bonemeal supplements should list the calcium and phosphorus levels per tablet or per teaspoon (5 mL) on the label. If that information is not supplied, contact the manufacturer. The information is necessary to ensure that you are adding the appropriate level of nutrients.

When adding bonemeal to your dog's diet, find the chart that corresponds to his/her weight (see pages 198 to 207). This chart shows the approximate amounts of naturally occurring calcium and phosphorus present in the sample recipe and the dog's minimum daily requirements (set by the National Research Council). It is recommended that the bonemeal supplement itself meets the NRC's minimum requirements for calcium and phosphorus in the charts. As noted, supplement half that amount, twice a day.

Multivitamin-and-Mineral Supplement

To ensure that your dog receives the full range of vitamins and minerals s/he needs, in addition to bonemeal, you will need to add a multivitamin-and-mineral supplement to his/her diet. The nutrient levels provided by the supplement should be included on the package label.

When adding a multivitamin-and-mineral supplement, find the chart that corresponds to your dog's weight (see pages 198 to 207). This chart shows the approximate amounts of naturally occurring vitamins and minerals present in the sample recipe and the dog's minimum daily requirements (set by the National Research Council). It is recommended that the multivitamin-and-mineral supplement itself meets or gets fairly close to the NRC's minimum requirements in the charts. Supplement half that amount twice a day.

> ### Tip
> Many pet multivitamin-and-mineral supplements are designed for use with commercial dog foods that already contain added vitamins and minerals. As a result, they have fairly low nutrient levels. Be sure to look for a product that is suitable for use with a home-prepared diet (i.e., that has moderately higher levels of nutrients than most other supplements). The supplement should meet or get fairly close to the NRC's minimum requirements. If you can't find an appropriate pet supplement, consult your pharmacist regarding use of one intended for humans. Such a tablet may need to be divided or doubled, depending on the size of your dog.

Toxicity Levels of Vitamins and Minerals

SOME OF THE ESSENTIAL VITAMINS AND MINERALS ARE toxic at a certain level. However, in most cases, there is a fairly wide margin of error.

These maximum nutrient levels are based upon units per 1,000 kcal ME (metabolizable energy, or the energy available in food that is ultimately used by the tissues).

Minerals

Calcium	7.1 g
Phosphorus	4.6 g
Magnesium	0.86 g
Iron	857 mg
Copper	71 mg
Zinc	286 mg
Iodine	14 mg
Selenium	0.57 mg

Vitamins

Vitamin A	71,429 IU
Vitamin D	1,429 IU
Vitamin E	286 IU

* toxicity levels for other nutrients were not addressed, as they may not be of concern due to contributing factors.

Sourced from the *2002 Official Publication*, Association of American Feed Control Officials Incorporated, © 2002.
For more information or to purchase a copy of the AAFCO 2002 Official Publication, please contact:
  Ms. Sharon Senesac, AAFCO Assistant Secretary-Treasurer,
  P.O. Box 478, Oxford, IN, 47971.
  Telephone: (765)-385-1029. E-mail: sharon@localline.com

Minimum Vitamin and Mineral Requirements by Weight

THE FOLLOWING CHARTS WILL PROVIDE THE INFORMATION you need to choose supplements that meet your dog's requirements. When using these charts, bear in mind that your dog has specific nutritional needs that are related to his/her weight. While larger dogs need less energy per pound or kilogram of body weight, dogs' nutrient needs do not decrease accordingly. Always refer to the appropriate chart (pages 198 to 207) to find your dog's minimum nutrient requirements.

The following charts are based on information provided by the National Research Council's committee on animal nutrition. New information on canine nutrition is constantly emerging. To stay up-to-date on current information, check periodically with places such as the National Academy Press (http://www.nap.edu).

Notes

- Feed your dog two meals a day.
- Add half the daily supplementation at each meal.
- Sodium, potassium and chloride have been added to the recipes in the forms of iodized table salt and potassium chloride (salt substitute). As a dog's requirements for these nutrients will be met with the recipe, these minerals do not need to be considered when looking for a multivitamin-and-mineral supplement.

Key

- g= gram   1 gram (g) = 1,000 milligrams (mg)
- mg= milligram   1 milligram (mg) = 1,000 micrograms (µg)
- µg= microgram

NUTRIENT REQUIREMENTS OF A 5-LB | 2.3 KG DOG
(Based on a recipe providing 226 kcal)

	Recipe example approx values	Minimum requirements per day — NRC
Calcium (Ca)	28 mg	274 mg
Iron (Fe)	1.5 mg	1.49 mg
Magnesium (Mg)	50 mg	18.8 mg
Phosphorus (P)	144 mg	205 mg
Zinc (Zn)	2.7 mg	1.65 mg
Copper (Cu)	0.138 mg	0.138 mg
Manganese (Mn)	0.75 mg	0.23 mg
Iodine (I)	0.01 mg	0.028 mg
Selenium (Se)	16.4 µg	5 µg
Thiamin (B1)	100 µg	46 µg
Riboflavin (B2)	150 µg	115 µg
Niacin (B3)	3,400 µg	517 µg
Pantothenic Acid (B5)	430 µg	460 µg
Pyridoxine (B6)	250 µg	51 µg
Cyanocobalamin (B12)	0.9 µg	1.15 µg
Folic Acid	0 µg	9.2 µg
Choline	75 mg	58 mg
Vitamin A	3,878 IU	173 IU
Vitamin D	N/A	18.4 IU
Vitamin E	1.15 IU	1.15 IU

NUTRIENT REQUIREMENTS OF A 10-LB | 4.5 KG DOG
(Based on a recipe providing 370 kcal)

	Recipe example approx values	Minimum requirements per day — NRC
Calcium (Ca)	46 mg	536 mg
Iron (Fe)	2.5 mg	2.92 mg
Magnesium (Mg)	82 mg	36.9 mg
Phosphorus (P)	237 mg	401 mg
Zinc (Zn)	4.4 mg	3.24 mg
Copper (Cu)	0.22 mg	0.27 mg
Manganese (Mn)	1.2 mg	0.45 mg
Iodine (I)	0.03 mg	0.054 mg
Selenium (Se)	27 µg	9.9 µg
Thiamin (B1)	170 µg	90 µg
Riboflavin (B2)	250 µg	225 µg
Niacin (B3)	5,700 µg	1,013 µg
Pantothenic Acid (B5)	700 µg	900 µg
Pyridoxine (B6)	400 µg	99 µg
Cyanocobalamin (B12)	1.5 µg	2.25 µg
Folic Acid	0 µg	18 µg
Choline	123 mg	113 mg
Vitamin A	6,399 IU	338 IU
Vitamin D	N/A	36 IU
Vitamin E	1.8 IU	2.25 IU

NUTRIENT REQUIREMENTS OF A **15**-LB | **6.8** KG DOG
(Based on a recipe providing 475 kcal)

	Recipe example approx values	Minimum requirements per day — NRC
Calcium (Ca)	58 mg	809 mg
Iron (Fe)	3.2 mg	4.4 mg
Magnesium (Mg)	105 mg	56 mg
Phosphorus (P)	302 mg	605 mg
Zinc (Zn)	5.6 mg	4.89 mg
Copper (Cu)	0.29 mg	0.4 mg
Manganese (Mn)	1.6 mg	0.68 mg
Iodine (I)	0.03 mg	0.08 mg
Selenium (Se)	34 µg	15 µg
Thiamin (B1)	220 µg	136 µg
Riboflavin (B2)	310 µg	340 µg
Niacin (B3)	7,200 µg	1,530 µg
Pantothenic Acid (B5)	900 µg	1,360 µg
Pyridoxine (B6)	500 µg	150 µg
Cyanocobalamin (B12)	1.9 µg	3.4 µg
Folic Acid	0 µg	27 µg
Choline	157 mg	170 mg
Vitamin A	8,145 IU	510 IU
Vitamin D	N/A	54 IU
Vitamin E	2.4 IU	3.4 IU

NUTRIENT REQUIREMENTS OF A **20**-LB | **9.0** KG DOG
(Based on a recipe providing 615 kcal)

	Recipe example approx values	Minimum requirements per day — NRC
Calcium (Ca)	75 mg	1,071 mg
Iron (Fe)	4 mg	5.8 mg
Magnesium (Mg)	135 mg	74 mg
Phosphorus (P)	391 mg	801 mg
Zinc (Zn)	7.3 mg	6.5 mg
Copper (Cu)	0.37 mg	0.54 mg
Manganese (Mn)	2 mg	0.9 mg
Iodine (I)	0.06 mg	0.1 mg
Selenium (Se)	44 µg	20 µg
Thiamin (B1)	290 µg	180 µg
Riboflavin (B2)	410 µg	450 µg
Niacin (B3)	9,400 µg	2,025 µg
Pantothenic Acid (B5)	1,000 µg	1,800 µg
Pyridoxine (B6)	700 µg	198 µg
Cyanocobalamin (B12)	2.4 µg	4.5 µg
Folic Acid	0 µg	36 µg
Choline	203 mg	225 mg
Vitamin A	10,540 IU	675 IU
Vitamin D	N/A	72 IU
Vitamin E	3.1 IU	4.5 IU

NUTRIENT REQUIREMENTS OF A **25**-LB | **11.3** KG DOG
(Based on a recipe providing 714 kcal)

	Recipe example approx values	Minimum requirements per day — NRC
Calcium (Ca)	88 mg	1,345 mg
Iron (Fe)	4.8 mg	7.3 mg
Magnesium (Mg)	158 mg	93 mg
Phosphorus (P)	456 mg	1,006 mg
Zinc (Zn)	8.5 mg	8.1 mg
Copper (Cu)	0.43 mg	0.68 mg
Manganese (Mn)	2.4 mg	1.1 mg
Iodine (I)	0.06 mg	0.13 mg
Selenium (Se)	52 µg	25 µg
Thiamin (B1)	340 µg	226 µg
Riboflavin (B2)	470 µg	565 µg
Niacin (B3)	10,900 µg	2,542 µg
Pantothenic Acid (B5)	1,300 µg	2,260 µg
Pyridoxine (B6)	800 µg	249 µg
Cyanocobalamin (B12)	2.8 µg	5.6 µg
Folic Acid	0 µg	45 µg
Choline	237 mg	282 mg
Vitamin A	12,273 IU	847 IU
Vitamin D	N/A	90 IU
Vitamin E	3.6 IU	5.6 IU

NUTRIENT REQUIREMENTS OF A **30**-LB | **13.6** KG DOG
(Based on a recipe providing 803 kcal)

	Recipe example approx values	Minimum requirements per day — NRC
Calcium (Ca)	99 mg	1,618 mg
Iron (Fe)	5.4 mg	8.8 mg
Magnesium (Mg)	177 mg	111 mg
Phosphorus (P)	512 mg	1,210 mg
Zinc (Zn)	9.6 mg	9.8 mg
Copper (Cu)	0.49 mg	0.81 mg
Manganese (Mn)	2.7 mg	1.4 mg
Iodine (I)	0.06 mg	0.16 mg
Selenium (Se)	58 µg	30 µg
Thiamin (B1)	380 µg	272 µg
Riboflavin (B2)	530 µg	680 µg
Niacin (B3)	12,300 µg	3,060 µg
Pantothenic Acid (B5)	1,500 µg	2,720 µg
Pyridoxine (B6)	900 µg	299 µg
Cyanocobalamin (B12)	3.2 µg	6.8 µg
Folic Acid	0 µg	54 µg
Choline	266 mg	340 mg
Vitamin A	13,784 IU	1,020 IU
Vitamin D	N/A	109 IU
Vitamin E	4 IU	6.8 IU

NUTRIENT REQUIREMENTS OF A **35**-LB | **15.8** KG DOG
(Based on a recipe providing 888 kcal)

	Recipe example approx values	Minimum requirements per day — NRC
Calcium (Ca)	110 mg	1,880 mg
Iron (Fe)	6 mg	10.2 mg
Magnesium (Mg)	197 mg	130 mg
Phosphorus (P)	569 mg	1,406 mg
Zinc (Zn)	10.7 mg	11.4 mg
Copper (Cu)	0.54 mg	0.95 mg
Manganese (Mn)	3 mg	1.6 mg
Iodine (I)	0.06 mg	0.19 mg
Selenium (Se)	65 µg	35 µg
Thiamin (B1)	420 µg	316 µg
Riboflavin (B2)	590 µg	790 µg
Niacin (B3)	13,600 µg	3,555 µg
Pantothenic Acid (B5)	1,700 µg	3,160 µg
Pyridoxine (B6)	1,000 µg	348 µg
Cyanocobalamin (B12)	3.6 µg	7.9 µg
Folic Acid	0 µg	63 µg
Choline	296 mg	395 mg
Vitamin A	15,315 IU	1,185 IU
Vitamin D	N/A	126 IU
Vitamin E	4.5 IU	7.9 IU

NUTRIENT REQUIREMENTS OF A **40**-LB | **18.1** KG DOG
(Based on a recipe providing 1,045 kcal)

	Recipe example approx values	Minimum requirements per day — NRC
Calcium (Ca)	129 mg	2,154 mg
Iron (Fe)	7.1 mg	11.8 mg
Magnesium (Mg)	231 mg	148 mg
Phosphorus (P)	666 mg	1,611 mg
Zinc (Zn)	12.5 mg	13 mg
Copper (Cu)	0.64 mg	1.09 mg
Manganese (Mn)	3.5 mg	1.8 mg
Iodine (I)	0.11 mg	0.22 mg
Selenium (Se)	76 µg	40 µg
Thiamin (B1)	500 µg	362 µg
Riboflavin (B2)	700 µg	905 µg
Niacin (B3)	16,000 µg	4,073 µg
Pantothenic Acid (B5)	2,000 µg	3,620 µg
Pyridoxine (B6)	1,200 µg	398 µg
Cyanocobalamin (B12)	4.2 µg	9 µg
Folic Acid	0 µg	72 µg
Choline	346 mg	452 mg
Vitamin A	17,919 IU	1,357 IU
Vitamin D	N/A	145 IU
Vitamin E	5.3 IU	9 IU

NUTRIENT REQUIREMENTS OF A **45**-LB | **20.4** KG DOG
(Based on a recipe providing 1,078 kcal)

	Recipe example approx values	Minimum requirements per day — NRC
Calcium (Ca)	133 mg	2,428 mg
Iron (Fe)	7.3 mg	13.2 mg
Magnesium (Mg)	238 mg	167 mg
Phosphorus (P)	686 mg	1,816 mg
Zinc (Zn)	12.8 mg	14.7 mg
Copper (Cu)	0.65 mg	1.2 mg
Manganese (Mn)	3.6 mg	2 mg
Iodine (I)	0.11 mg	0.24 mg
Selenium (Se)	78 µg	45 µg
Thiamin (B1)	510 µg	408 µg
Riboflavin (B2)	720 µg	1,020 µg
Niacin (B3)	16,500 µg	4,590 µg
Pantothenic Acid (B5)	2,000 µg	4,080 µg
Pyridoxine (B6)	1,200 µg	449 µg
Cyanocobalamin (B12)	4.3 µg	10.2 µg
Folic Acid	0 µg	82 µg
Choline	357 mg	510 mg
Vitamin A	18,473 IU	1,530 IU
Vitamin D	N/A	163 IU
Vitamin E	5.4 IU	10.2 IU

NUTRIENT REQUIREMENTS OF A **50**-LB | **22.6** KG DOG
(Based on a recipe providing 1,164 kcal)

	Recipe example approx values	Minimum requirements per day — NRC
Calcium (Ca)	143 mg	2,689 mg
Iron (Fe)	7.9 mg	14.7 mg
Magnesium (Mg)	256 mg	185 mg
Phosphorus (P)	740 mg	2,011 mg
Zinc (Zn)	13.8 mg	16.2 mg
Copper (Cu)	0.71 mg	1.3 mg
Manganese (Mn)	3.8 mg	2.3 mg
Iodine (I)	0.11 mg	0.27 mg
Selenium (Se)	84 µg	50 µg
Thiamin (B1)	550 µg	452 µg
Riboflavin (B2)	770 µg	1,130 µg
Niacin (B3)	17,700 µg	5,085 µg
Pantothenic Acid (B5)	2,200 µg	4,520 µg
Pyridoxine (B6)	1,300 µg	497 µg
Cyanocobalamin (B12)	4.6 µg	11.3 µg
Folic Acid	0 µg	90 µg
Choline	384 mg	565 mg
Vitamin A	19,910 IU	1,695 IU
Vitamin D	N/A	181 IU
Vitamin E	5.8 IU	11.3 IU

NUTRIENT REQUIREMENTS OF A **60**-LB | **27.2** KG DOG
(Based on a recipe providing 1,334 kcal)

	Recipe example approx values	Minimum requirements per day — NRC
Calcium (Ca)	165 mg	3,237 mg
Iron (Fe)	9.1 mg	17.7 mg
Magnesium (Mg)	296 mg	223 mg
Phosphorus (P)	854 mg	2,421 mg
Zinc (Zn)	16 mg	19.6 mg
Copper (Cu)	0.82 mg	1.6 mg
Manganese (Mn)	4.5 mg	2.7 mg
Iodine (I)	0.11 mg	0.33 mg
Selenium (Se)	97 µg	60 µg
Thiamin (B1)	640 µg	544 µg
Riboflavin (B2)	890 µg	1,360 µg
Niacin (B3)	20,500 µg	6,120 µg
Pantothenic Acid (B5)	2,500 µg	5,440 µg
Pyridoxine (B6)	1,500 µg	598 µg
Cyanocobalamin (B12)	5.3 µg	13.6 µg
Folic Acid	0 µg	109 µg
Choline	443 mg	680 mg
Vitamin A	22,973 IU	2,040 IU
Vitamin D	N/A	218 IU
Vitamin E	6.8 IU	13.6 IU

NUTRIENT REQUIREMENTS OF A **70**-LB | **31.7** KG DOG
(Based on a recipe providing 1,492 kcal)

	Recipe example approx values	Minimum requirements per day — NRC
Calcium (Ca)	184 mg	3,772 mg
Iron (Fe)	10.1 mg	20.6 mg
Magnesium (Mg)	330 mg	260 mg
Phosphorus (P)	951 mg	2,821 mg
Zinc (Zn)	17.8 mg	22.8 mg
Copper (Cu)	0.91 mg	1.9 mg
Manganese (Mn)	5 mg	3.2 mg
Iodine (I)	0.17 mg	0.38 mg
Selenium (Se)	108 µg	70 µg
Thiamin (B1)	710 µg	634 µg
Riboflavin (B2)	1,000 µg	1,585 µg
Niacin (B3)	22,800 µg	7,133 µg
Pantothenic Acid (B5)	2,800 µg	6,340 µg
Pyridoxine (B6)	1,700 µg	697 µg
Cyanocobalamin (B12)	6 µg	15.8 µg
Folic Acid	0 µg	127 µg
Choline	494 mg	792 mg
Vitamin A	25,598 IU	2,377 IU
Vitamin D	N/A	254 IU
Vitamin E	7.6 IU	15.8 IU

NUTRIENT REQUIREMENTS OF AN *80*-LB | *36.2* KG DOG
(Based on a recipe providing 1,658 kcal)

	Recipe example approx values	Minimum requirements per day — NRC
Calcium (Ca)	205 mg	4,308 mg
Iron (Fe)	11.3 mg	23.5 mg
Magnesium (Mg)	366 mg	297 mg
Phosphorus (P)	1,057 mg	3,222 mg
Zinc (Zn)	19.8 mg	26 mg
Copper (Cu)	1 mg	2.2 mg
Manganese (Mn)	5.5 mg	3.6 mg
Iodine (I)	0.17 mg	0.43 mg
Selenium (Se)	121 µg	80 µg
Thiamin (B1)	790 µg	724 µg
Riboflavin (B2)	1,100 µg	1,810 µg
Niacin (B3)	25,400 µg	8,145 µg
Pantothenic Acid (B5)	3,200 µg	7,240 µg
Pyridoxine (B6)	1,900 µg	796 µg
Cyanocobalamin (B12)	6.6 µg	18.1 µg
Folic Acid	0 µg	145 µg
Choline	549 mg	905 mg
Vitamin A	28,442 IU	2,715 IU
Vitamin D	N/A	290 IU
Vitamin E	8.4 IU	18.1 IU

NUTRIENT REQUIREMENTS OF A *90*-LB | *40.8* KG DOG
(Based on a recipe providing 1,776 kcal)

	Recipe example approx values	Minimum requirements per day — NRC
Calcium (Ca)	219 mg	4,855 mg
Iron (Fe)	12 mg	26.5 mg
Magnesium (Mg)	391 mg	334 mg
Phosphorus (P)	1,129 mg	3,631 mg
Zinc (Zn)	21.1 mg	29.3 mg
Copper (Cu)	1.1 mg	2.4 mg
Manganese (Mn)	5.9 mg	4.1 mg
Iodine (I)	0.17 mg	0.49 mg
Selenium (Se)	129 µg	90 µg
Thiamin (B1)	840 µg	816 µg
Riboflavin (B2)	1,200 µg	2,040 µg
Niacin (B3)	27,100 µg	9,180 µg
Pantothenic Acid (B5)	3,400 µg	8,160 µg
Pyridoxine (B6)	2,000 µg	898 µg
Cyanocobalamin (B12)	7.1 µg	20.4 µg
Folic Acid	0 µg	163 µg
Choline	586 mg	1,020 mg
Vitamin A	30,371 IU	3,060 IU
Vitamin D	N/A	326 IU
Vitamin E	8.9 IU	20.4 IU

NUTRIENT REQUIREMENTS OF A *100*-LB | *45.3* KG DOG
(Based on a recipe providing 1,971 kcal)

	Recipe example approx values	Minimum requirements per day — NRC
Calcium (Ca)	243 mg	5,391 mg
Iron (Fe)	13.4 mg	29.4 mg
Magnesium (Mg)	436 mg	371 mg
Phosphorus (P)	1,257 mg	4,032 mg
Zinc (Zn)	23.5 mg	32.6 mg
Copper (Cu)	1.2 mg	2.7 mg
Manganese (Mn)	6.6 mg	4.5 mg
Iodine (I)	0.23 mg	0.54 mg
Selenium (Se)	143 µg	100 µg
Thiamin (B1)	940 µg	906 µg
Riboflavin (B2)	1,300 µg	2,265 µg
Niacin (B3)	30,100 µg	10,192 µg
Pantothenic Acid (B5)	3,700 µg	9,060 µg
Pyridoxine (B6)	2,200 µg	997 µg
Cyanocobalamin (B12)	7.9 µg	22.6 µg
Folic Acid	0 µg	181 µg
Choline	653 mg	1,132 mg
Vitamin A	33,809 IU	3,397 IU
Vitamin D	N/A	362 IU
Vitamin E	10 IU	22.6 IU

NUTRIENT REQUIREMENTS OF A *110*-LB | *49.8* KG DOG
(Based on a recipe providing 2,090 kcal)

	Recipe example approx values	Minimum requirements per day — NRC
Calcium (Ca)	258 mg	5,926 mg
Iron (Fe)	14.2 mg	32.4 mg
Magnesium (Mg)	462 mg	408 mg
Phosphorus (P)	1,332 mg	4,432 mg
Zinc (Zn)	25 mg	35.8 mg
Copper (Cu)	1.28 mg	2.98 mg
Manganese (Mn)	7 mg	5 mg
Iodine (I)	0.23 mg	0.59 mg
Selenium (Se)	152 µg	109 µg
Thiamin (B1)	1,000 µg	996 µg
Riboflavin (B2)	1,400 µg	2,490 µg
Niacin (B3)	32,000 µg	11,205 µg
Pantothenic Acid (B5)	4,000 µg	9,960 µg
Pyridoxine (B6)	2,400 µg	1,096 µg
Cyanocobalamin (B12)	8.4 µg	24.9 µg
Folic Acid	0 µg	199 µg
Choline	692 mg	1,245 mg
Vitamin A	35,838 IU	3,735 IU
Vitamin D	N/A	398 IU
Vitamin E	10.6 IU	24.9 IU

NUTRIENT REQUIREMENTS OF A *120*-LB | **54.4** KG DOG
(Based on a recipe providing 2,271 kcal)

	Recipe example approx values	Minimum requirements per day — NRC
Calcium (Ca)	280 mg	6,474 mg
Iron (Fe)	15.4 mg	35.3 mg
Magnesium (Mg)	502 mg	446 mg
Phosphorus (P)	1,448 mg	4,842 mg
Zinc (Zn)	27.1 mg	39.1 mg
Copper (Cu)	1.39 mg	3.26 mg
Manganese (Mn)	7.6 mg	5.4 mg
Iodine (I)	0.23 mg	0.65 mg
Selenium (Se)	165 µg	120 µg
Thiamin (B1)	1,080 µg	1,088 µg
Riboflavin (B2)	1,500 µg	2,720 µg
Niacin (B3)	34,700 µg	12,240 µg
Pantothenic Acid (B5)	4,300 µg	10,880 µg
Pyridoxine (B6)	2,600 µg	1,197 µg
Cyanocobalamin (B12)	9.1 µg	27.2 µg
Folic Acid	0 µg	218 µg
Choline	752 mg	1,360 mg
Vitamin A	38,954 IU	4,080 IU
Vitamin D	N/A	435 IU
Vitamin E	11.5 IU	27.2 IU

NUTRIENT REQUIREMENTS OF A *130*-LB | **58.9** KG DOG
(Based on a recipe providing 2,375 kcal)

	Recipe example approx values	Minimum requirements per day — NRC
Calcium (Ca)	293 mg	7,009 mg
Iron (Fe)	16.1 mg	38.2 mg
Magnesium (Mg)	525 mg	483 mg
Phosphorus (P)	1,514 mg	5,242 mg
Zinc (Zn)	28.4 mg	42.4 mg
Copper (Cu)	1.45 mg	3.5 mg
Manganese (Mn)	7.9 mg	5.9 mg
Iodine (I)	0.23 mg	0.70 mg
Selenium (Se)	173 µg	130 µg
Thiamin (B1)	1,100 µg	1,178 µg
Riboflavin (B2)	1,600 µg	2,945 µg
Niacin (B3)	36,300 µg	13,252 µg
Pantothenic Acid (B5)	4,500 µg	11,780 µg
Pyridoxine (B6)	2,700 µg	1,296 µg
Cyanocobalamin (B12)	9.5 µg	29.4 µg
Folic Acid	0 µg	236 µg
Choline	786 mg	1,472 mg
Vitamin A	40,725 IU	4,417 IU
Vitamin D	N/A	471 IU
Vitamin E	12 IU	29.4 IU

NUTRIENT REQUIREMENTS OF A *140*-LB | *63.4* KG DOG
(Based on a recipe providing 2,488 kcal)

	Recipe example approx values	Minimum requirements per day — NRC
Calcium (Ca)	307 mg	7,545 mg
Iron (Fe)	16.9 mg	41.2 mg
Magnesium (Mg)	550 mg	520 mg
Phosphorus (P)	1,586 mg	5,643 mg
Zinc (Zn)	29.7 mg	45.6 mg
Copper (Cu)	1.5 mg	3.8 mg
Manganese (Mn)	8.3 mg	6.3 mg
Iodine (I)	0.23 mg	0.76 mg
Selenium (Se)	181 µg	139 µg
Thiamin (B1)	1,200 µg	1,268 µg
Riboflavin (B2)	1,600 µg	3,170 µg
Niacin (B3)	38,000 µg	14,265 µg
Pantothenic Acid (B5)	4,700 µg	12,680 µg
Pyridoxine (B6)	2,800 µg	1,395 µg
Cyanocobalamin (B12)	10 µg	31.7 µg
Folic Acid	0 µg	254 µg
Choline	824 mg	1,585 mg
Vitamin A	42,664 IU	4,755 IU
Vitamin D	N/A	507 IU
Vitamin E	12.6 IU	31.7 IU

NUTRIENT REQUIREMENTS OF A *150*-LB | *68.0* KG DOG
(Based on a recipe providing 2,679 kcal)

	Recipe example approx values	Minimum requirements per day — NRC
Calcium (Ca)	331 mg	8,092 mg
Iron (Fe)	18.2 mg	44.2 mg
Magnesium (Mg)	592 mg	558 mg
Phosphorus (P)	1,708 mg	6,052 mg
Zinc (Zn)	32 mg	48.9 mg
Copper (Cu)	1.6 mg	4.0 mg
Manganese (Mn)	8.9 mg	6.8 mg
Iodine (I)	0.23 mg	0.81 mg
Selenium (Se)	195 µg	150 µg
Thiamin (B1)	1,300 µg	1,360 µg
Riboflavin (B2)	1,800 µg	3,400 µg
Niacin (B3)	41,000 µg	15,300 µg
Pantothenic Acid (B5)	5,100 µg	13,600 µg
Pyridoxine (B6)	3,000 µg	1,496 µg
Cyanocobalamin (B12)	10.7 µg	34 µg
Folic Acid	0 µg	272 µg
Choline	887 mg	1,700 mg
Vitamin A	45,946 IU	5,100 IU
Vitamin D	N/A	544 IU
Vitamin E	13.5 IU	34 IU

Resources

Chapter 1

Articles

Bren, Linda. "Pet Food: The Lowdown on Labels," *FDA Consumer* 35, no. 3 (May-June 2001).
http://www.fda.gov/fdac/features/2001/301_pet.html

Dzanis, David A. "Vegetarian Diets For Pets?" *FDA Veterinarian Newsletter* 24, no. 111 (May-June 1999).
http://www.fda.gov/cvm/index/fdavet/1999/may.html#vegetarian

Freeman, Lisa M., and Kathryn E. Michel. "Evaluation of Raw Food Diets for Dogs," *Veterinary Medicine Today: Timely Topics in Nutrition, Journal of the American Veterinary Medical Association* 218, no. 5 (2001): 705–709.

Homsey, Christine M. "Phytochemicals: Beyond Vitamins and Minerals," *Food Product Design* (July 1999).
http://www.foodproductdesign.com/archive/1999/0799cs.html

Horowitz, Janice M. "10 Foods that Pack a Wallop," *Time*, January 21, 2002, 51–55.

Joffe, Daniel J., and Daniel P. Schlesinger. "Preliminary Assessment of the Risk of Salmonella Infection in Dogs Fed Raw Chicken Diets," *The Canadian Veterinary Journal* 43 (June 2002): 441–442.

Patil, A.R., and G.C. Fahey, Jr. "Pet Food Ingredients and Ingredient Processing Affect Dietary Protein Quality," in *Proceedings, 1998 Purina Nutrition Forum, Supplement to Compendium on Continuing Education for the Practicing Veterinarian* 21, no. 11(k) (November 1999).

Web Sites

Canadian Food Inspection Agency (1-800-442-2342)
http://www.inspection.gc.ca

Dr. Ian Billinghurst
http://www.drianbillinghurst.com

United States Food and Drug Administration
http://www.fda.gov

Johnson, Jane. "Barf FAQ," Barfers.com (2000).
http://www.barfers.com/barf.html

Books

AAFCO 2002 Official Publication (Oxford, IN: Association of
   American Feed Control Officials Incorporated, 2002).

•••

Chapter 2

Articles

Broadhurst, C. Leigh. "The Essential PUFA Guide for Dogs and
   Cats," *Nutrition Science News* (October 2001).
   http://www.newhope.com/nutritionsciencenews/
   NSN_backs/Oct_01/pufa.cfm

Burger, Ivan H. "Assessing Needs of Companion Animals," *Journal of
   Nutrition* 124 (1994): F 2584–F 2593.

Burger, Ivan H., and Janel V. Johnson. "The Allometry of Energy
   Requirements Within a Single Species," *Journal of Nutrition* 121
   (1991): F 18–F 21.

"Nutritional Effects On Musculoskeletal Development."
   http://education.vetmed.vt.edu/Curriculum/VM8264/
   04/index.html

Stauth, David. "Dietary Oils Shown to Suppress Immune System,"
   Oregon State University News & Communication Services.
   http://orst.edu/dept/ncs/newsarch/1997/May97/dogoils.htm

Web Sites

Dogs — Basic Principles of Nutrition. Waltham Center for
   Pet Nutrition (2001).
   http://www.waltham.com/dogs/nutritional_science/
   basic_principles.html

Waltham Center for Pet Nutrition
   http://www.waltham.com

USDA Nutrient Database for Standard Reference, Release 14. U.S.
   Department of Agriculture, Agricultural Research Service (2001).
   http://nal.usda.gov/fnic/foodcomp

Books

AAFCO 2002 Official Publication (Oxford, IN: Association of
   American Feed Control Officials Incorporated, 2002).

Committee on Animal Nutrition, National Research Council.
   Nutrient Requirements of Dogs, Revised 1985 (Washington, D.C.:
   National Academy Press, 1985).
   http://www.nap.edu/books/0309034965/html/

Health Canada. *Nutrient Value of Some Common Foods*
   (Ottawa: 1999).

Kirschmann, John D., and Lavon J. Dunne. *Nutrition Almanac: Second Edition* (New York: McGraw-Hill, 1984).

Schoen, Allen M., and Susan G. Wynn. *Complementary and Alternative Veterinary Medicine: Principles and Practice* (St. Louis: Mosby, Inc., 1998).

Strombeck, Donald R. *Home-Prepared Dog and Cat Diets: The Healthful Alternative* (Ames, IA: Iowa State University Press, 1999).

••

Chapter 3

Articles

Food Safety and Inspection Service, United States Department of Agriculture. "Food Safety Facts Information for Consumers" (2001).
http://www.fsis.usda.gov/OA/pubs.facts_basics.htm

Magnuson, Bernadine. "Natural Toxins in Food Plants," Extoxnet FAQs (1997).
http://ace.orst.edu/info/extoxnet/faqs/natural/plant1.htm

Web Sites

ASPCA Animal Poison Control Center (1-888-426-4435)
http://apcc.aspca.org

Books

Birchard, Stephen J., and Robert G. Sherding. *Saunders Manual of Small Animal Practice* (Philadelphia: W.B. Saunders Co., 1994).

Dodman, Nicholas. *The Dog Who Loved Too Much: Tales, Treatments, and the Psychology of Dogs* (New York: Bantam Books, 1996).

Nesbitt, Gene H., and Lowell J. Ackerman. *Canine and Feline Dermatology: Diagnosis and Treatment* (Trenton: Veterinary Learning Systems, 1998).

Schoen, Allen M., and Susan G. Wynn. *Complementary and Alternative Veterinary Medicine: Principles and Practice* (St. Louis: Mosby, Inc., 1998).

The Merck Veterinary Manual, 7th Edition (New Jersey: Merck and Co., Inc., 1991).

Chapter 7

Committee on Animal Nutrition, National Research Council. *Nutrient Requirements of Dogs, Revised 1985* (Washington, D.C.: National Academy Press, 1985).

Additional References

Web Sites
Edwards, Geraint. "Vegetarian Glossary," Vegetarian Pages.
  http://old.veg.org/veg/FAQ/Glossary.html

Canola Council of Canada (204) 982-2100
  http://www.canola-council.org

Hall, Rick. About Nutrition (2002).
  http://nutrition.about.com/library/blvitamins.htm

POS Pilot Plant Corporation. "Comparison of Dietary Fats," Canola Council of Canada (1994).
  http://canola-council.org/pubs/fatcharts/english.html

The Truths and Myths About Canola. Canola Council of Canada (1999).
  http://www.canolainfo.org/htm/truth.html

Books
Carlson, Delbert G., and James M. Giffon. *Dog Owner's Home Veterinary Handbook: Revised and Expanded* (New York: Howell Book House, 1992).

Kalnins, Diana, and Joanne Saab. *Better Baby Food* (Toronto: Robert Rose Inc., 2001).

Pitcairn, Richard H., and Susan H. Pitcairn. *Dr. Pitcairn's Complete Guide to Natural Health for Dogs and Cats* (Emmaus City: Rodale Press Inc., 1995).

Thurston, Mary E. *The Lost History of the Canine Race: Our 15,000-Year Love Affair with Dogs* (Kansas City: Andrews and McMeel, 1996).

Volhard, Wendy, and Kerry Brown. *Holistic Guide for a Healthy Dog: Second Edition* (Foster City: Howell Book House, 2000).

Reading List

....

Behavior and Training

Coren, Stanley. *The Intelligence of Dogs: A Guide to the Thoughts, Emotions, and Inner Lives of Our Canine Companions* (New York: Bantam Books, 1995).

Dodman, Nicholas. *Dogs Behaving Badly: An A to Z Guide to Understanding & Curing Behavioral Problems in Dogs* (New York: Bantam Books, 1999).

Dodman, Nicholas. *The Dog Who Loved Too Much: Tales, Treatments, and the Psychology of Dogs* (New York: Bantam Books, 1996).

Eisenmann, Charles P. *Stop! Sit! and Think* (New York: MacDonald Redmore Inc., 1968).
Authors' Note: This book may be difficult to find, but it's well worth the effort if you are able to track a copy down.

Fox, Michael W. *Superdog: Raising the Perfect Canine Companion* (New York: Howell Book House, 1996).

Kilcommons, Brian, and Michael Capuzzo. *Mutts America's Dogs: A Guide to Choosing, Loving, and Living with Our Most Popular Canine* (New York: Warner Books, 1996).

Kilcommons, Brian, and Sarah Wilson. *Childproofing Your Dog: A Complete Guide to Preparing Your Dog for the Children in Your Life* (New York: Warner Books, 1994).

Kilcommons, Brian, and Sarah Wilson. *Good Owners, Great Dogs: A Training Manual for Humans and Their Canine Companions* (New York: Warner Books, 1992).

Any of the books, booklets or videos from Dr. Ian Dunbar.

Authors' Note: Training should be a positive experience for the dog and for the person. There are many humane training and therapy programs and resource guides available that can help people and their dogs deal with behavior problems. One outstanding service available to help with behavior problems is the Petfax consulting service. This service is provided by the Tufts Behavior Clinic at the Tufts University of Veterinary Medicine and is accessible to anyone, anywhere in the world. The Tufts Behavior Clinic can help with a vast range of problems, from minor issues to the most severe ones. For information about the Petfax service and prices, call (508) 839-8738 or visit the Web site at www.tufts.edu/vet/petfax/index.html.

Natural Diets and Health

Bamberger, Michelle. *Help! The Quick Guide to First Aid for Your Dog* (New York: Howell Book House, 1993).

Carlson, Delbert G., and James M. Giffon. *Dog Owner's Home Veterinary Handbook: Revised and Expanded* (New York: Howell Book House, 1992).

Goldstein, Martin. *Nature of Animal Healing: The Path to Your Pet's Health, Happiness, and Longevity* (New York: Alfred A. Knopf, 1999).

Martin, Ann M. *Food Pets Die For: Shocking Facts About Pet Food* (Troutdale: New Sage Press, 1997).

Pitcairn, Richard H., and Susan H. Pitcairn. *Dr. Pitcairn's Complete Guide to Natural Health for Dogs & Cats* (Emmaus City: Rodale Press Inc., 1995).

Strombeck, Donald R. *Home-Prepared Dog and Cat Diets: The Healthful Alternative* (Ames, IA: Iowa State University Press, 1999).

Various Topics

Kilcommons, Brian, and Sarah Wilson. *Paws to Consider: Choosing the Right Dog for You and Your Family* (New York: Warner Books, 1999).

Marshal Thomas, Elizabeth. *The Hidden Life of Dogs* (New York: Pocket Star Books, 1993).

Masson, Jeffrey Mousaieff. *Dogs Never Lie About Love: Reflections on the Emotional World of Dogs* (New York: Three Rivers Press, 1997).

Read, Nicholas. *One in a Million* (Vancouver: Polestar Sirius Books, 1996).
Authors' Note: This is a great story for children and adults, which teaches compassion for abandoned dogs.

Thurston, Mary E. *The Lost History of the Canine Race: Our 15,000-Year Love Affair with Dogs* (Kansas City: Andrews and McMeel, 1996).

Authors' Note: These are just a few of the many exceptional books that have been written about dogs. We encourage you to read as much as you can and to never stop learning.

Library and Archives Canada Cataloguing in Publication

Bastin, David
    Better food for dogs : a complete cookbook & nutrition guide / David Bastin,
Jennifer Ashton and Grant Nixon.

Includes index.
ISBN 978-0-7788-0424-6

    1. Dogs—Food—Recipes. 2. Dogs—Nutrition. 3. Dogs—Diseases—Diet therapy.
I. Ashton, Jennifer II. Nixon, Grant III. Title.

SF427.4.B38 2012   636.7'0852   C2012-902810-X

Index

M